Part 1
Pediatric pathologies

>>> Sous-partie 1 - Évaluation d'une détresse chez l'enfant

>>> Sous-partie 2 - Pathologies respiratoires

>>> Sous-partie 3 - Pathologies cardiaques

>>> Sous-partie 4 - Pathologies neurologiques

>>> Sous-partie 5 - Traumatologie

>>> Sous-partie 6 - Autres

Sub-Part 1
Assessment of a distress in the child

>>> Mémo 1 - Constantes et scores

>>> Mémo 2 - Prise en charge de la douleur

Memo

The Constants and Scores

Summary of the memo

1. Apgar score (D')
2. Burns: calculation of the surface
3. Glasgow (score)
4. Blood Glucose Levels: Standards
5. laryngitis: score of gravity
6. Malinas (score)
7. with multisystem trauma: referral to a trauma center
8. Silverman (score)

The CONSTANTS/Vital Signs

		0-1 month	1 months-2 years	2-4 years	4-10 years	> 10 years
Cf/min	Limits	90-180	80-155	70-140	59-113	55-105
	Prevent	< 90 or > 190	< 80 or > 170	< 70 or > 160	< 60 or > 140	< 50 or > 130

FR/min	To Normal	40	30	20	18	15
	Prevent	< 20 or > 60	< 15 or > 40	< 15 or > 30	< 10 or > 30	
SpO2 % in Air	Prevent	< 90		< 92		< 94
Pile mmHg	Limits	70-90	85-105	90-110	95-115	110-130
	Prevent	< 60 or > 100	< 75 or > 110	< 80 or > 130	< 85 or > 140	< 90 or > 160
TAD mmHg	Limits		40-60	50-65	55-70	65-80
TAM	Limits		45-55	65-80	70-	80

	mmHg				85 - 95	
	Prevent	< 45	< 60	< 65	< 70	< 80
Diuresis, ml/kg/h	To Normal	2-3		2	1-2	
	Prevent	< 1 or > 4 on 3 h			< 1 or > 4 on 6 h	

SpO2 : Acceptable values after the birth for SpO2 Sus ductale

2 minutes	60%
3 minutes	70%
4 minutes	80%
5 minutes	85%
10 minutes	90%

Hemodynamic distress of the Child

In the new-born in the first days of life	Beyond the 1 year
TA Average = term in (weeks of amenorrhea)	• Systolic blood pressure = 90 + [2 × Age (year)] • Hypo ta < 70 + [2 × Age (year)]

Tachycardia is the first sign of shock in children.

I ♦ Apgar score (D')

APGAR Virginia: physician anaesthetist-responder, 1909-1974.
Measured at 1 minute, 3 minutes, 5 minutes, 10 minutes.

Coloring	Blue Trunk or pale	0
	Pink trunk Blue ends	1
	Trunk and pink ends	2
Breathing	No	0
	Superficial	1
	Vigorous	2

	cry		
Tonus	Hypotonia	0	
	Means	1	
	Vigorous	2	
Reactivity **	No	0	
	Low	1	
	Vive	2	
Cardiac frequency	0	0	
	< 100	1	
	> 100	2	
		Total	/10

** Reactivity: spontaneous motor, Cree, sneezing, cough.

The Apgar score does not guide more the Resuscitation (ILCOR 2010, 2015), but has a prognostic value (see Mémo 34 Réanimation du nouveau-né).

• Apgar score > 7 : Normal, all goes well.
• Apgar Score < 3 : Poor adaptation to the extrauterine life, requires a resuscitation of the newborn.
• Apgar score between 3 and 7 : requires a supported specific.

II ♦ Burns: calculation of the surface
Among the child, the "Rule of 9" does not apply.

Determination of the surface burned

Location	0-1 year	1-4 years	5-9 years	10-15 years	Adult
The head	19%	17%	13%	10%	7%
Neck	2%	2%	2%	2%	2%
Anterior torso	13%	13%	13%	13%	13%
Posterior torso	13%	13%	13%	13%	13%
Buttock (each)	2.5%	2.5%	2.5%	2.5%	2.5%
The genitalia ext.	1%	1%	1%	1%	1%
Arm (each)	4%	4%	4%	4%	4%
Forearm (each)	3%	3%	3%	3%	3%
Hand (each)	2.5%	2.5%	2.5%	2.5%	2.5%
Thigh (each)	5.5%	6.5%	8.5%	8.5%	9.5%
Leg (each)	5%	5%	5.5%	6%	7%
Foot (each)	3.5%	3.5%	3.5%	3.5%	3.5%

SFETB 1992

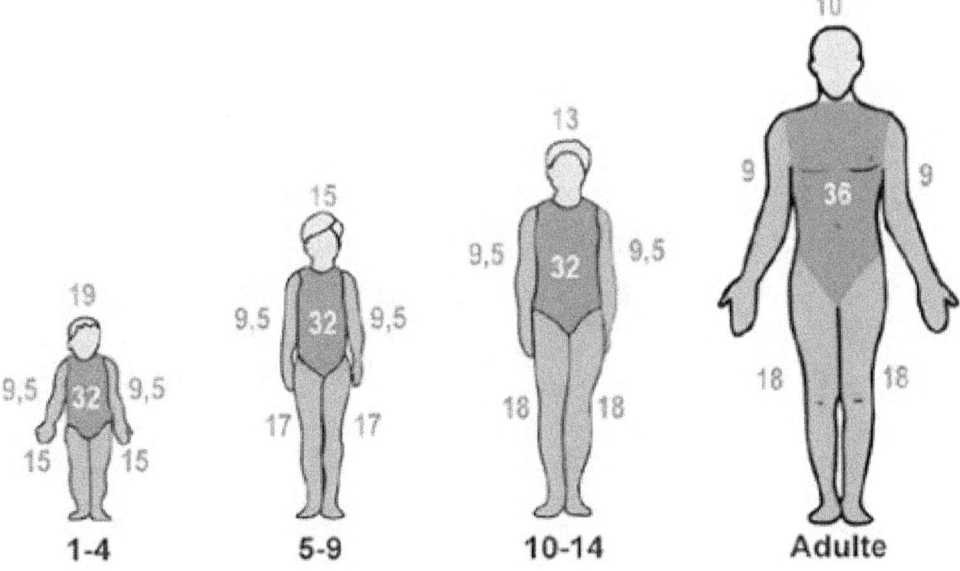

It can also calculate the burned surface using the surface of the palm of the hand of the patient who represents 1 per cent of the body surface area.

Attention!
• Before the burns of the face and neck = **intubation in emergency** except for burns by hot liquid.
• Before any burning of the perineum = **urinary probe in emergency.**

III ♦ Glasgow (score)

♦ Glasgow adult and large child

Opening the eyes = Y	Spontaneous	4
	To the order	3
	To pain	2
	No	1

Verbal response = V	Oriented	5
	Confused	4
	Inappropriate	3
	Incomprehensible	2
	No	1
Motor response = M	Obeys the simple Order	6
	Oriented to the PAIN	5
	Non-oriented to the PAIN	4
	Decorticate	3
	Pithing	2
	No	1

• Glasgow Coma Score ≤ 8 = Intubation
• But in préhospitalier, it must always weigh the benefit risk.

The method of nociceptive stimulation Validated is the pressure supported at sus-orbital or the pressure of the nail bed with a pen. The friction or pinching of the skin should be avoided.

♦ **Pediatric Glasgow**

Opening the eyes	Spontaneous	4	
	At the request	3	
	To pain	2	
	No	1	
	Verbal response	Social behavior	5
		Consolables crying	4
		Incessant Cree	3
		Agitation, moans	2
		No	1
		Best motor response	Spontaneous movements	6
			Withdraws to the touch	5
			Withdraws to pain	4
			Decorticate, abnormal bending	3

		Pithing, abnormal extension	2
		No	1

IV ♦ Blood Glucose Levels: Standards

Age	Low value	High Value
New-born	2.2 mmol/L (0.4 g/L)	11 mmol/l (2 g/L)
Child	3.3 mmol/L (0.6 g/L)	7 mmol/l (1.26 g/L)

V ♦ laryngitis: score of gravity

	Minor	Moderate	Severe
Hoarse coughing	Occasional basis	Frequent	Frequent
Stridor at rest	Absent	This	Present at the inspiration and expiration
Draw sus-stermal/ Intercostal drawing	Absent or minimal	At rest	Marked
Agitation, disturbances of	Absent	Absent or minimal	This

consciousness			

Alberta Clinical Practice Guideline Working Group, 2008

VI ♦ Malinas (score)
Allows you to quickly assess the risk of a imminent delivery.

Parity	1	0				
	2	1				
	3 And More	2				
	Duration of work	< 3 h	0			
		Between 3 and 5 h	1			
		> 5 h	2			
		Duration of contraction	< 1 min	0		
			1 min	1		
			> 1 min	2		
			Duration between contractions	> 5 min	0	
				Between 3 and 5 min	1	
				< 3 min	2	
				Loss of	Non	0

water	Recent	1
	> 1 h	2
	Total	/10

• Score of Malinas < 5 → transport not medicalized in CWD to the nearest maternity facility.

• Score of Malinas > 5 → imminent delivery.
• Factor accelerating : want to push.

♦ Criterion of medicalization
• Score of Malinas.
• Remoteness, duration of transport.
• Pathology associated (HTA, twins, seat...).

VII ♦ with multisystem trauma: referral to a trauma center

Lesion mechanism	• Ejection of a vehicle.
	• A passenger on the same vehicle died.
	• Fall of more than 6 meters.
	• Projected victim or crushed.
	• Kinetics (deformation of the vehicle, estimated speed, lack of helmet or seat belt).
	• Blast.
Physiological criteria	• Disorder of the conscience.
	• Vital distress.

Anatomical criteria	• Pediatric Trauma Score < 8.
	• Penetrating trauma or amputation.
	• Chest trauma severe.
	• Abdominal defense.

♦ *Pediatric Trauma Score (PTS)*

The Pediatric Trauma Score (PTS) is a tool to estimate the risk of death during a trauma in pediatrics. It takes into account the specificities of the physiology of the Child by integrating the weight and the state of the airway in the calculation.

The minimum score is - 6 and the maximum is + 12. The more the PTS is low, the more the risk of mortality is high (estimated risk to 100% if score ≤ 0), the more the PTS is high, the more the risk of mortality is low (estimated risk to 9% if score ≥ 8).

	+ 2	+ 1	- 1
Weight	> 20 kg	10-20 kg	< 10 kg
The airway	Free	With assistance	Required intubation
Systolic blood pressure	> 90 mmHg	50-90 mmHg	< 50 mmHg
The Glasgow Coma Score	15-12	11-9	≤ 8
The fractures	No	Closed	Multiple open/
Wounds	No	Minimal	Major

VIII ♦ Silverman (score)

→ mnemonic : Baby (Swaying/beat) derives (draw) in (funnel) Geignant (geignement).

Swinging thoraco-abdominal	Absent	0
	Stationary chest	1
	Paradoxical breathing	2
Draw	Absent	0
	Discreet intercostal	1
	+ intercostal sus- and sub-sternal	2
Xypholdien funnel	Absent	0
	Moderate	1
	Intense	2

Beat of wings of the nose	Absent	0
	Moderate	1
	Intense	2
Respiratory geignement	Absent	0
	Collected at the stethoscope	1
	Audible at the ear in continuous	2
	Total	/10

Score of severity: Silverman > 4

Memo 2
Support for the pain

I ♦ Definition
According to the International Association for the Study of Pain (IASP): Pain is a sensory and emotional experience associated unpleasant to tissue damage real or potential.

The Act of 4 March 2002, on the Rights of the sick and to the quality of the health system stipulates that "any person has the right to receive care aimed to relieve his pain. The latter must be in any circumstance prevented, evaluated, taken into account and treated."

II ♦ Evaluation

A. A few notions of the perception of pain in the child
• From 0 to 2 years : sensation of comprehensiveness of the painful act, not of understanding, anticipation of relief.

• 2 to 7 years : there is no link between the cause and the consequence, children often associate two events (white coats = stitching). The pain is experienced as a punishment. This is the age where the child think the pain may disappear by magic.

• From 7 to 11 years : stage of concrete operations, ability to establish a relationship between the pain and the disease. The children are in capacity to describe the pain and quantify.

• Among Adolescents : they are able to express their fears, they are able to understand the disease, its evolution, its treatments.

These concepts are important in order to establish a relationship of trust with the child by associating it with a supported medication: make knowledge with the child, to observe, discuss, exchange with the parents prior to assess the pain.

B. The scales are most used in the Pediatrics

There are several scales of assessment. They are chosen by the caregiver as a function of the age of the Child:
- < 7 years: hetero-assessment;
- > 7 years Self-assessment.

♦ For the hetero-assessment
• EVENDOL Scale : Scale used to emergencies and in préhospitalier among children from birth to 7 years. It allows to assess any type of pain simply and quickly. The threshold of treatment is reached from a rating of 4/15.

→ see _tableau_ next page.

♦ For the self-assessment
• Digital Scale, also called "Scale of Faces ": allows the child to move the cursor on the face which expresses the pain felt (" chosen the face that shows how much Thou hast poorly at this time. ").
• Scale EVS : rating of the pain of 0 to 4.

♦ Other scales used in a specific context

• EDIN, Dan for the Neonatology, of the premature until the infant to 3 months :
- The Edin evaluates the prolonged pain and discomfort thanks to the observation of the items: face, body, sleep, relationship, comfort. The score is 0 to 15, the threshold of pain treatment is done from a score of 5.
- The scale Dan evaluates the acute pain through the observation of 3 items: Face, movements, crying. The score is 0 to 10, the threshold of pain treatment is done from 2.

• Comfort-B, for patients sédatés : it allows to assess the pain and sedation. It is used in préhospitalier, in resuscitation and post-operative. The score is 6 to 30. The threshold of allows rating to determine if the child is too sédaté, comfortable, in a state border with a possible pain or clearly uncomfortable.

• FLACC, for the post-operative, and FLACC amended, adapted to the evaluation of the acute pain in a child in a situation of disability : it can be used from birth to 18 years (19 years in the case of a disability). The rating for each item is done from 0 to 2. The score is between 0 and 10.

EVENDOL

Evaluation Enfant Douleur

Echelle validée de la naissance à 7 ans.
Score de 0 à 15, seuil de traitement 4/15

Notez tout ce que vous observez... même si vous pensez que les signes ne sont pas dus à la douleur, mais à la peur, à l'inconfort, à la fatigue ou à la gravité de la maladie.

Nom	Signe absent	Signe faible ou passager	Signe moyen ou environ la moitié du temps	Signe fort ou quasi permanent	Evaluation à l'arrivée		Evaluations suivantes / Evaluations après antalgique							
					au repos ou calme (R)	à l'examen¹ ou la mobilisation (M)	R	M	R	M	R	M	R	M
Expression vocale ou verbale														
pleure et/ou crie et/ou gémit et/ou dit qu'il a mal	0	1	2	3										
Mimique														
a le front plissé et/ou les sourcils froncés et/ou la bouche crispée	0	1	2	3										
Mouvements														
s'agite et/ou se raidit et/ou se crispe	0	1	2	3										
Positions														
a une attitude inhabituelle et/ou antalgique et/ou se protège et/ou reste immobile	0	1	2	3										
Relation avec l'environnement														
peut être consolé et/ou s'intéresse aux jeux et/ou communique avec l'entourage	normale 0	diminuée 1	très diminuée 2	absente 3										
	Score total /15													
	Date et heure													
Remarques					Initiales évaluateur									

¹ Au repos ou calme (R) : observer l'enfant avant tout soin ou examen, dans les meilleures conditions possibles de confort et de confiance, par exemple à distance, avec ses parents, quand il joue...
² A l'examen ou la mobilisation (M) : il s'agit de l'examen clinique ou de la mobilisation ou palpation de la zone douloureuse par l'infirmière ou le médecin.
Réévaluer régulièrement en particulier après antalgique, au moment du pic d'action : après 30 à 45 minutes si oral ou rectal, 5 à 10 minutes si IV. Préciser la situation, au repos (R) ou à la mobilisation (M)

Echelle validée pour mesurer la douleur (aiguë ou prolongée, nociceptive, avec ou sans composante neuropathique) de 0 à 7 ans, en présence ou en l'absence de soignant, au SAMU, en salle de réveil, en post-opératoire... Références bibliographiques : Archives de Pédiatrie 2009 ;13 :922 ; 17(9)1350, Archives de Pédiatrie 2011 ;19 :622, PA2644, Journées Paris Pédiatrie 2009 ;285,358, Pain 2012 ;153 :1573-1582. Contact : elisabeth.fournier-charriere.aphp.fr © 2011 Groupe EVENDOL

III ♦ Processing

A. Anticipate the pain of care

♦ anesthésiante cream (lidocaine and prilocaine)

Dose : Premature between 30 and 37 weeks, a hazelnut of 0.5 g on a single site, once a day, 1 h Maximum time to install (outside AMM).

Age	Posology	Application Time
0-2 months	1 g	1 h
3-11 months	2 g	1 h
1-5 years	10 g	1-5 h
6-11 years	20 g	1-5 h

Technical :
* Tube or skin patch.
* Apply the cream in thick layer without spread (hazelnut) and cover it with an adhesive bandage of type TEGADERM®, if available use directly the anaesthetic patch already packaged.
* Always note the time of the installation.
* Wipe off the cream before the care.

♦ sweet solution to referred pain reliever (sucrose solution 24%)

Dose : effectiveness among the new-born and the infant up to 4-6 months. The associate to the suction not nutritious, to care containers, to the Cream anesthésiante.

Weight	Posology
< 1 000 g	1 to 2 drops (0.05 to 0.1 ml)

Of 1 000 g to 1 500 g	3 to 4 drops (0.15 to 0.2 ml)
Of 1 000 g to 2 000 g	5 to 7 drops (0.25 to 0.35 ml)
≥ 2 000 g	8 to 10 drops (0.4 to 0.5 ml)
Maximum 6 to 8 times per day	

Technical :
* Administer on the language, drip, using a syringe. The analgesic effect appears 1-2 minutes after the administration and has a duration of action of 5-7 minutes.
* Renew the administration if the care lasts for more than 5 minutes.

♦ Nitrous Oxide

Equimolar mixture of oxygen (50%) and nitrous oxide (50%). It is a colorless and odourless gas. It is a anxiolytic and analgesic surface, to use in association with the Cream anesthésiante, methods of distraction and/or other treatments analgesics.

Contraindications :
- Head trauma, intracranial hypertension;
- Alteration of the state of consciousness;
- Pneumothorax;
- Bubble of emphysema;
- Gaseous embolism;
- Abdominal distension, PNEUMOPERITONEUM;
- Facial trauma;
- Known deficit and not substituted for vitamin B12.

Dose and Technical:
* To breathe the gas 3 minutes to the child that it begins to act.
* Continue the inhalation during the entire duration of the Act.
* The balloon present on the system of inhalation should never be collabé, it must adapt the gas flow by function.

♦ distraction and hypnoanalgésie

• In pediatrics, a special place will be made for parents, reassure, their explain the conduct of the care.
• Use of the ^{means of distraction} (games, lint, songs) to appease the child during care and transport (Unknown location, medical staff).
• Mobilize parents as ^{resource persons, ask them if the child has a Doudou and take knowledge of its centers of interest.}
• The hypnoanalgésie is a method of increasingly widespread and used in préhospitalier, notably pediatrics to take in charge the anxiety and pain of the Child (in association with drug means).

>>> **Examples of distraction by the game (stuffed toys, soft toys)**

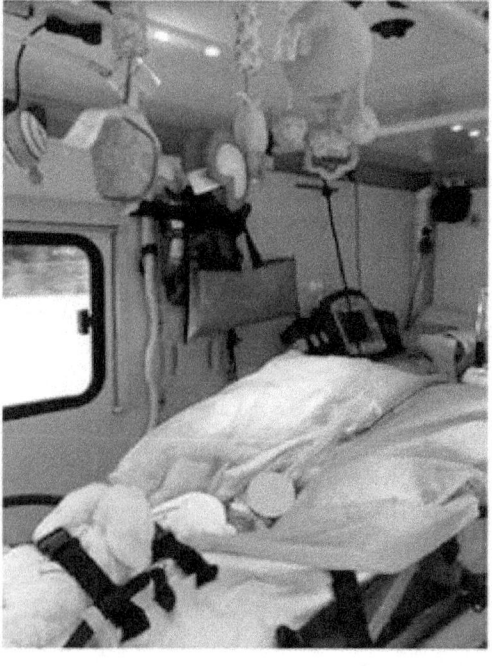
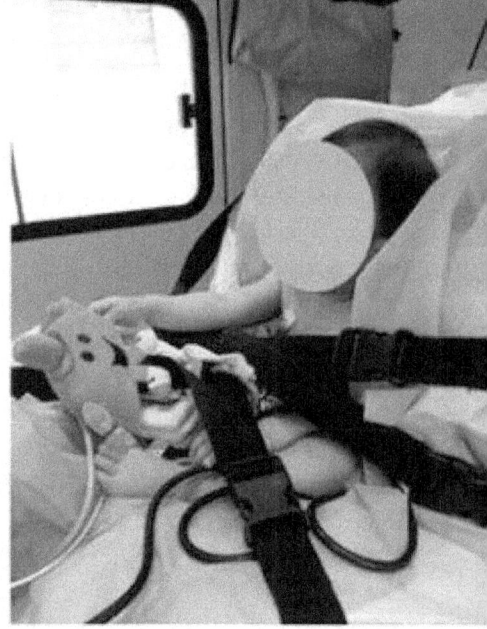

© A.M./N.L.

B. Supported medicinal products

Level I	Mild pain	• Paracetamol
		• Non-steroidal anti-inflammatory drug
		• Néfopam (> 15 years)
Tier II	Moderate pain	• Codeine (> 12 years)
		• Destropropoxyphène
		• Tramadol (> 3 years)
Level III	Intense pain	• Morphine
		• Fentanyl
		• Opioid derivatives

• Paracetamol : analgesic and antipyretic activity.
IV : 15 mg/kg.
PO : 15 mg/kg/6 h.
• Ibuprofen : non-steroidal anti-inflammatory drug.
PO : 10 mg/kg/8 h.
• Nalbuphine : central analgesic semi-synthetic type of agonist/morphine antagonist of the series of phenanthrenes.
IV : 0.2 mg/kg/4 h or 1.2 mg/kg/i in IV continues, delay in Action 2-3 minutes.
IR : 400 mcg/kg or 0.4 mg/kg, delay of action 10-15 minutes.

• Morphine Sulfate : ORAMORPH®.
Single-dose container of 10 mg/5 ml.
PO : 1 mg/kg/day max. dose 20 mg.
< 5 kg = 0.1 mg/kg/socket.
> 5 kg = 0.5 mg/kg in dose of load and then titration of 0.2 mg/kg/30 min. up to effectiveness and then equivalent to the total dose received by titration (without the dose of load)/4 h.
• Morphine : opioid analgesic.
IV :
- Loading dose: 50-100 mcg/kg,

- Then 25 mcg/kg in titration.

Maintenance : 20-40 mcg/kg/h.
• Ketamine : general anaesthetic.
Sedation/analgesia:
IV : 0.2 to 0.5 mg/kg.
IR : 5-10 mg/kg.
Time limit for action : 60 seconds.
Duration of action : 5-15 minutes.

→ *For indications and contra-indications refer to the fact sheets Pharmacology (see Partie 4).*

Think About It

The acceptance of the pain of the Premature is recent: For years, it was denied because of the idea of the immaturity of the receivers, of nerve pathways and myelination incomplete.

To this day, **the perception of the pain of the Premature is no longer to demonstrate. The latter has an immediate effect in the new-born premature (apneas, increase oxygen requirements, tachycardia or bradycardia, increased stress, discomfort, poor digestion etc.). This is why it is necessary to limit the number of painful gestures, organize the care, consolidate the levies, reduce nuisances and promote to the maximum the presence of parents.**

Sub-Part 2
Respiratory diseases

>>> Mémo 3 - Asthme

>>> Mémo 4 - Bronchiolite

>>> Mémo 5 - Dyspnée

>>> Mémo 6 - Épiglottite

>>> Mémo 7 - Inhalation d'un corps étranger

>>> Mémo 8 - Laryngite

Memo 3
Asthma

I ♦ Definition
Asthma is a chronic inflammatory disease of the Airways with a bronchial obstruction reversible and hypersecretion of mucus causing acute dyspnea.

♦ aggravating elements
• < 4 years or adolescent.
• Asthma Former, unstable, already 1 Stay in resuscitation, recent hospitalization.
• Respiratory Infection.
• Obesity.

II ♦ Signs
The signs are of a sudden onset or may be preceded by a prodrome of viral respiratory infection.
The wheezing.

♦ signs of seriousness
• Crisis of asthma unusual and rapid evolution and progressive.
• Inability to speak, orthopnea, dyspnoea at rest.
• Respiratory rate > 40/min (2 to 5 years), > 30/min (> 5 years).
• Restlessness.
• Sweating, cyanosis.
• Normo or hypercapnia.
• Hypotension (TA < to 2 standard deviations in relation to the age).
• SpO2 in vs < 90%.

♦ signs of distress
• Auscultation silent.
• Respiratory depletion or extreme tachypnea (FR + 50 per cent compared to the age).
• Respiratory pauses.
• Disorders of the conscience.

• Bradycardia, hypotension.

• Hypercapnia.

III ♦ Supported in préhospitalier
• Installation in a half-sitting position (do not lengthen the child: risk of cab).
• Oxygen therapy if need, aim SpO2 > 94%.
• Monitoring (FR, FC, NBP, SpO2).
• Measurement of the blood glucose levels.
• Measurement of the temperature.
• Install VVP if necessary.
• Re-evaluation of the clinical condition after each therapeutic intervention, and fundamental reassessment to 60 minutes.
• The extent of the DEP is not a priority in context préhospitalier. It can be conducted in the child > 6 years of age who does not present signs of severe respiratory distress (risk of worsening and delays in processing).
• Transport medicalized, hospitalization in the ICU systematic if severe crisis, or as soon as the administration of magnesium sulfate or salbutamol IV.

IV ♦ Processing

♦ The β2 (inhaled salbutamol, terbutaline)
• Nebulization classic with O2 6 to 8 l/min.
• Spray + House of inhalation: salbutamol : 1 puff/3 kg (min. : 2 puffs, max. : 10 puffs).
Method of administration:
- < 18 months: 10 respi with the House of inhalation after each puff;
- > 18 months: 5 Respi after each puff. Repeat two times this treatment with a 20-min interval between doses.
• Salbutamol in nebulization:
- 2.5 mg/nébul. for < 20 kg;
- 5 mg/nébul. For the > 20 kg.
• Or terbutaline in nebulization: 1 drop/kg/nébul (min. = 8 drops, max. = 1 POD = 5 mg).
• Salbutamol or in continuous nebulization for the severe crises: 0.45 mg/kg/h (min. : 1.5 mg/h, max. : 15 mg/h).

• Association with ipratropium bromide and systemic corticosteroids.

♦ systemic corticosteroid (for crisis slight to severe)
• Anti-inflammatory: increases the sensitivity to the β2. Must be administered quickly because noticeable effect in 6 to 12 h.
• No difference IV or per os in the child.
• Betamethasone 0.05% Po: 20 drops/kg or 0.25 mg/kg.
• Or prednisolone PO : 1 to 2 mg/kg.
• Or methylprednisolone IV: 1 mg/kg.

Anticholinergic ♦ (for the moderate crises/severe)
• Ipratropium Bromide
• Synergistic Action with the β2.
• Ipratropium bromide in nebulization (paediatric dose): 0.25 mg/nébul.
Administer concomitantly with Beta-2, a treatment on two. Can be put in the same nebulizer as salbutamol/terbutaline.

♦ Magnesium Sulfate
• 25 to 40 mg/kg of the sulphate of Mg in 20 min.
• Side effects: vasoplégie, hypotension, disorders of the pace.
• Should be attempted before the addition of salbutamol IV.

♦ β2 IV
Extreme gravity or insufficient response to treatment
• Salbutamol iv: 0.5 to 5 mcg/kg/min ; If the relay treatment in continuous nebulization, begin to 2 mcg/kg/min.
• Stop the treatment in nebulization of β2.
• Side effects: tremor, tachycardia, hypokalemia, cardiac toxicity rare among the child.

♦ The NAV
More and more used by some teams of resuscitation for the support of acute asthma very severe. It could be considered in some patients to prevent intubation. It is a field in full evolution.

♦ Intubation

Intubation is a treatment of last resort. The mechanical ventilation of a patient in acute asthma is complex and at high risk of complications.
* Indications of intubation (orotrachea, sit to balloon tip):
- ACR;
- Major hypoxemia;
- Rapid degradation of the conscience;
- Insufficient decompensated respiratory;
- Worsening under treatment well led.
* Intubation in rapid sequence:
- Atropine (for the drainage of secretions): 20 mcg/kg;
- Ketamine (bronchodilator): 2 to 4 mg/kg;
- Not of local anesthesia to lidocaine ;
- Curarisation;
- Consider a filling at the physiological serum pre or per-intubation, because collapses of PCA frequent.

Mechanical ventilation avoiding the dynamic hyperinflation at the price of a permissive hypercapnia (up to pH = 7.10) but ensuring a correct oxygenation.

Current Volume 5 to 6 ml/kg

Pressure plate = 30 cm H20 (max. 40)

Ratio of I/E: 1/3, Ti Min 0.5 s

Frequency 8 to 12/min

PEEP = 0 initially

- Need for a effective sedation;
- Sometimes, curarisation necessary, prefer bolus of curare long action to the infusion.

♦ **treatment of last resort**

* **External compression of the thoracic cage** during the expiry, in ventilation at the Bavu.
* Instillation intra-tracheal of adrenaline 10 mcg/kg or salbutamol 5 mg.
* Transitional Use of a PEP. According to the recommendation.
* Assistance extracorporeal respiratory (areca nut).

V ♦ Decision Tree

Severe crisis	Moderate crisis	Mild crisis
Rare sibilants	Sibilants +/- cough	Sibilants +/- cough
Vesicular murmur decreased or absent	FR increased	Normal FR
Nurse distress franche + cyanosis	Implementation of the respiratory muscles Accessories	No respiratory distress, not of cyanosis
Activity impossible	Walking difficult	Activity and Floor
Slurred speech	Whispers 2 to 3 words	Normal speech
Fall PA Systolic/Diastolic		
Low response to ß2	Answer kept in the ss2	Answer kept in the ss2
DEP ≤ 50%	50% < DEP < 75%	DEP > 75%

| SpO2 ≤ 90% | 90% < SpO2 < 95% | SpO2 ≥ 95% |

>>> Treatment of acute asthma of the Child

- Position demi-assise.
- Ne pas allonger l'enfant (risque d'ACR).
- Oxygénothérapie si besoin pour SpO_2 > 94 %.
- Monitoring.
- Pose de VVP si nécessaire.

1) β2 inhalés
- Salbutamol : 1 bouffée/3 kg. Min 2 bouffées - max 10 bouffées.
- Salbutamol en nébulisation : 2,5 mg si < 20 kg, 5 mg si > 20 kg.
- OU terbutaline en nébulisation : 1 goutte/kg, minimum 8 gouttes.
- Salbutamol en nébulisation continue pour les cas sévères : 0,45 mg/kg/h (min 1,5 mg/h, max 15 mg/h).

1) Corticothérapie systémique
Effet perceptible 6/12 h, à administrer rapidement.
- Betamethasone 0,05 % PO : 20 gouttes/kg soit 0,25 mg par kg.
- OU prednisolone PO : 1 à 2 mg/kg.
- OU methylprednisolone IV : 1 mg/kg.

2) Anticholinergique : si crise modérée ou sévère
- Bromure d'Ipratropium en nébulisation : 0,25 mg < 20 kg, 0,5 mg > 20 kg.
- Administrer de façon concomitante avec les Beta 2 un traitement sur deux.

3) Sulfate de magnésium
- Dose : 25 à 40 mg/kg de sulfate de Mg en 20 min.
- Attention à l'hypotension.

4) β2 IV
- Salbutamol : 0,5 à 5 mcg/kg/min, débuter à 2 mcg/kg/min si en relais d'une nébulisation continue.

5) Intubation à séquence rapide et ventilation
après remplissage sérum physiologique 20 ml/kg.
- Atropine : 20 mcg/kg.
- Kétamine : 2 à 4 mg/kg.
- Curarisation.
Sédation +/- curarisation

→ Volume Courant 5 à 6 ml/kg
Pression plateau = 30 cm H_2O (max 40)
Ratio I/E : 1/3, Ti min 0,5 sec
Fréquence 8 à 12/min
PEEP = 0 initialement

6) Traitement de dernier recours
- Compression externe de la cage thoracique pendant l'expiration, en ventilation à l'AMBU.
- Instillation intra trachéale d'adrénaline 10 mcg/kg ou de salbutamol 5 mg.
- Utilisation transitoire d'une PEP élevée.
- AREC

Memo 4
Bronchiolitis

I ♦ Definition
Viral infection epidemic respiratory seasonal (winter context) Beginner by acute nasopharyngitis, then reaching the lower respiratory tract. The respiratory syncytial virus is the etiologic agent in 70% of cases.

II ♦ Signs
Clinics: sibilants and wheezing and/or sub-crépitants.

♦ form well tolerated
- FR < 60/min.
- SpO2 > 95%.
- Respiration wide.
- Good reactivity.
- Power supply not disrupted.

♦ signs of seriousness
- Respiratory distress:
Rapid Shallow Breathing -;
- Signs of a struggle;
- Respiratory depletion;
- Apnea;
- Cyanosis or desaturation with SpO2 < 91% under 3-5 L/Min O2 nasal;
- Respiratory acidosis.
- Congestion of the respiratory tract.
- Tachycardia and/or decrease in peripheral perfusion/Central.
- Grayish complexion.
- Decrease in the tone.
- Difficulty in feeding.
- Vomiting or diarrhea.
- Hyperthermia.

* Alteration of the state of consciousness.
* Collapse.

♦ aggravating elements
* Infants < 6 weeks.
* Former premature < 34 SA and < 3 months of age corrected.
* Bronchodysplasie.
* Congenital Heart Disease/PAH.
* Immunocompromised.

III ♦ Supported in préhospitalier
* Unblocking rhino-pharyngeal (DRP).
* Buccal aspirations nasopharyngeal and.
* Proclive.
* Monitoring (FR, FC, SpO2, NIBP, signs of a struggle).
* Measurement of the blood glucose levels.
* Measurement of the temperature.
* O2 for SpO2 ≥ 94%
* Assess the need for a track IV if sign of seriousness important or sign of dehydration and supply difficult.

IV ♦ Processing
→ If form well tolerated, treatment at home:
- Education of Parents (DRP);
- Inform the parents on the signs of worsening that can induce a hospitalization;
- Respiratory kiné urgent in city, 2/J if congestion.
→ If sign of seriousness or need for O2 maintain SpO2 ≥ 94%, transportation to SAU.
If a support by ventilatory NIV or intubation is necessary, the patient will be transferred to a resuscitation service pediatric.
* **Niv:** very effective in the Support for acute bronchiolitis.
Indications of NIV:
- Apneas;
- Worsening of signs of struggle or sign of respiratory depletion;
- Need to O2 > 2 l/min in nasal glasses to maintain ≥ 94%.
Niv with VS-PEP + 7 and FiO2 for a saturation ≥ 94%. The use of a heater humidifier is desirable;

- Interface via binasale cannula or nasal mask maintained by a hat or a harness; usefulness of the nipple to close the mouth (less leaks);
- Monitoring of the SpO2, FR, FC and if possible the TcPCO2;
- The criteria of effectiveness of the NIV are a decline in the FR, of the CF and the TcPCO2, and an improvement of the SpO2 in the 2 hours following the installation of the VNI.

•**Intubation:** Since the introduction of the NIV in the treatment of bronchiolitis, recourse to intubation is less and less frequent.
Indications of intubation:
- Failure of the NIV after 2 to 4 h of establishment;
- Severe hypoxemia despite NIV;
- Frequent apneas and/or severe despite VNI.

Think About It

Before a shallow breathing in epidemic period, namely, evoke a heart failure linked to a myocarditis before making a diagnosis too fast of bronchiolitis.

Memo 5
Dyspnea

I ♦ Definition
Dyspnea is a difficulty or an embarrassment to the respiration that can be appreciated on the different time respiratory. It can be accompanied by a modification of the respiratory rhythm: Shallow breathing or bradypnée. The cause of the Dyspnoea may be respiratory, infectious disease, cardiac, metabolic or mechanical.

II ♦ Signs
• Respiratory rate: Shallow breathing/bradypnée.
• Irregularity of the respiratory frequency.
• Superficial breathing.

♦ signs of seriousness
• Severity of the signs of respiratory distress or signs of respiratory depletion.
• Respiratory rate < 10 or > 60 cycles/min.

• Tachycardia.

• Sweating.

• Disorders of the Conscience, loss of contact with parents or caregivers.

• Restlessness.

• Hypotonia.

• Total obstruction of the airways.
• Pallor or cyanosis.

♦ signs of a struggle
Intercostal draw or sub-costal, circulation, sus-clavicular, rocking thoraco-abdominal, beat of the wings of the nose, xyphoïdien funnel, expiratory geignement, head bobbing (use sternocleidomastoid muscles).

III ♦ Supported in préhospitalier

Respiratory insufficiency offset	Respiratory insufficiency Decompensated
• Assess	• Assess
• Position of comfort	• Open the airway
• O2 if necessary	• Monitoring (FC-FR-SpO2-NBP)
• Monitoring (FC-FR-SpO2-NBP)	• O2 100%
• Measurement of the blood glucose	• Measurement of the blood glucose
• Measurement of the temperature	• Measurement of the temperature
• Give nothing per os except medication	• To assist the ventilation if necessary (NAV)
• Track IV if necessary	• Consider intubation + mechanical ventilation
• Specific Treatment	• Specific Treatment
• Regularly reevaluate	• Reassess
	• Admission to resuscitation service
	• Assess if resource in ORL necessary

IV ♦ Processing
Supported in drug function of the etiology.

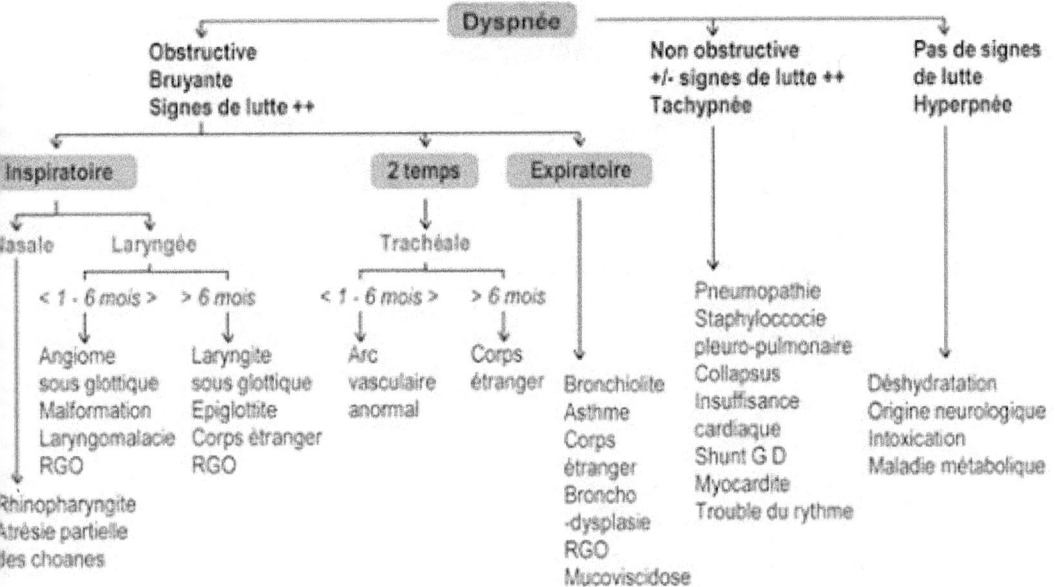

Memo 6
Epiglottitis

I ♦ Definition
Bacterial infection and inflammation of the Epiglottis, sudden onset and of rapid evolution. Historically caused by Haemophilus influenzae type B.

II ♦ Signs

♦ Epidemiology
* Average age: 3 years.
* Seasonal Peak (fall-winter).

♦ signs of seriousness
* Child sitting refusing any other position (to respect +++ Otherwise risk of cab).
* Hypoxia (gray complexion, cyanosis, pallor).
* Inspiratory Dyspnea without cough with stridor.
* Voice stifled.
* Hypercapnia.
* Draw sus-sternal and sus-clavicular.
* Hyperthermia ≥ 40o.
* Lymphadenopathy The submaxillary+++.
* Hypersialorrhée.

♦ signs of distress
* Respiratory Disorders with apneas.
* Exhaustion.
* Collapse.

III ♦ Supported in préhospitalier

* Respect the sitting position - do not look at the Throat = risk of ACR.

• Take contact with a surgical block or a room of alarm clock with ENT specialty paediatric (if possible) to practice intubation by fibroscopie upon arrival. Ensure a place in resuscitation service for the result of the supported.
• Put the child in confidence, do not cry, promote to the maximum the presence of parents.

● Monitoring.

• Install VVP desirable, but transport without venous access to consider if patient stable and hospital receiver nearby to avoid a respiratory decompensation during the care.
• O2 if necessary.
• Quick Transfer in a seated position.

IV ♦ Processing
• Injection of 50 mg/kg of cefotaxime IV.
• If IV impossible, Ceftriaxone 50 mg/kg IM (thigh).
• Nebulization of 5 mg of adrenaline, renew if necessary.

Think About It

Think of the epiglottitis in children not vaccinated against Haemophilus influenzae b.

Memo 7
Inhalation of a foreign body

I ♦ Definition
A syndrome of bronchial penetration may occur when the inhalation of a foreign body. It may stay at the level of the glottis, space sub-glottal, of the trachea or a bronchus causing a violent coughing with asphyxiation. The child must be transferred to a hospital with ENT specialty paediatric (if possible).

II ♦ Signs

♦ signs of partial obstruction
- Restlessness.
- Cough.
- Wheezing.
- The child bears the hands to his throat.
- Partial incapacity to express themselves.

♦ signs of total obstruction
- Cough not effective or not cough.
- Breathing impossible.
- Total incapacity to express themselves.
- Cyanosis.
- Disorders of the conscience.

III ♦ Supported in préhospitalier
- Monitoring (cf, FR, NBP, SpO2).
- If partial obstruction:
- A half-sitting position;
- Put the child in confidence, do not cry, promote to the maximum the presence of parents;
- Oxygen if necessary to maintain SpO2 ≥ 94%;

- Install VVP desirable, but transport without venous access to consider if patient stable and hospital receiver nearby to avoid respiratory decompensation during the care;
- Transfer in ORL (pediatric if possible).

• *If total obstruction:* See *point 5 – Arbre décisionnel*

IV ♦ Processing

♦ method of Mofenson (adapted to children < 1 year)
* Look in the mouth if a foreign body is visible.
* If the foreign body is visible, unclog manually using a bracketed finger, or a compresses.
* Return the child and the chock astride the forearm supporting it on the knee, head tilted down, keep the mouth of the child opened with two fingers between the corners of the lips.
* With the palm of the hand, practice 5 tapes farms between the shoulder blades.
* If the foreign body is not expelled, return the child face to itself and make 5 chest compressions (with two fingers 1 cm below the line mamelonnaire).
* Repeat the operation (Alternate 5 pats on the back / 5 chest compressions) up to expulsion of foreign body or until the child falls unconscious.

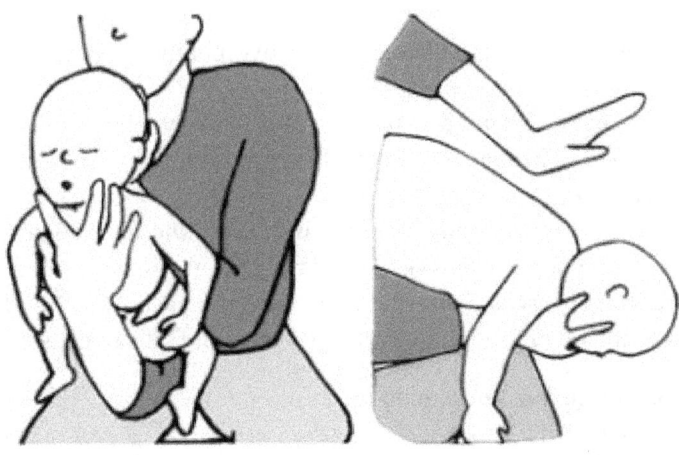

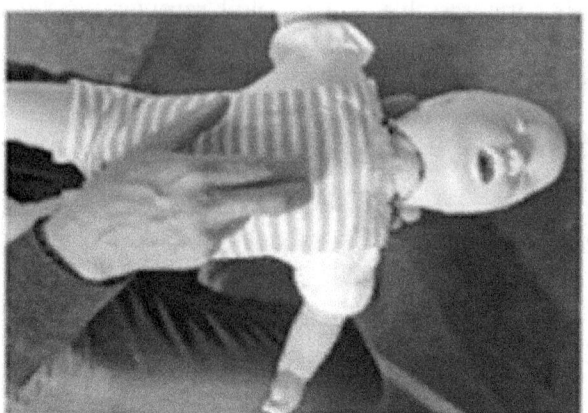

© L.D.

♦ method of Heimlich (adapted for children > 1 year)
* Look in the mouth if a foreign body is visible.
* If the foreign body is visible, unclog manually using a bracketed finger, or a compresses.
* Position themselves on the side of the Child, the leaning slightly toward the front in the supporting of a hand.
* Using the palm of the hand, giving 5 tapes farms between the shoulder blades.
* If the foreign body is not expelled, move behind the child, wrap the Arm around him.
* Close the fist of a hand and put two fingers above the navel, at the level of the diaphragm. Place the other hand on top of the point to be used as a lever.
* Compress 5 times firmly toward the top of the abdominal wall (pull in exercising a pressure toward the rear and upwards).
* Repeat the operation (Alternate 5 pats on the back / 5 HEIMLICH) up to expulsion of foreign body or until the child falls unconscious.

♦ In case of unconsciousness
* Open the airway.
* Practice 5 breaths, and then begin cardiopulmonary resuscitation.

• Opportunity to push back the foreign body in the bronchus right strain during intubation (to remove in a second time by endoscopy).

♦ **If failure**
Cricothyroïdotomie of fortune: see Mémo 42.

V ♦ Decision Tree

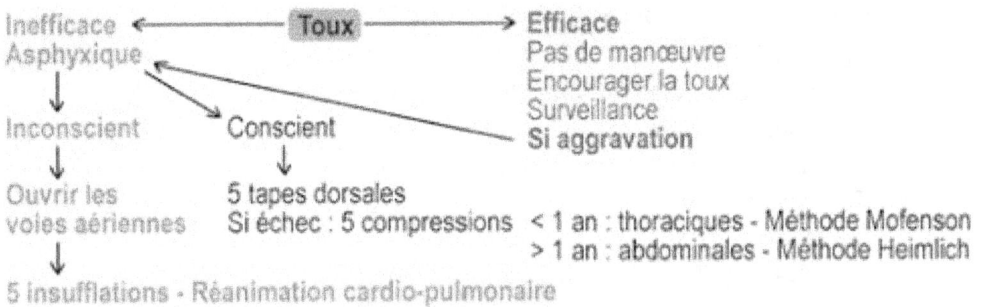

Memo 8

Laryngitis

I ♦ Definition
Acute inflammation of the sub-glottis by viral infection. Inspiratory dyspnea of sudden onset. Occurred at night.

II ♦ Signs
• Laryngeal dyspnoea with Inspiratory stridor. The stridor may not be present that to the crying in the case of slight laryngitis or present at rest in the case of moderate laryngitis.
• Tachypnea.
• Voice off or raspy.
• Hoarse coughing spasmodic,.

♦ signs of seriousness
• Drowsiness.
• Stridor at rest.
• Tachycardia.
• Draw sus-sternal and sus-clavicular, printing of asphyxiation.
• Mild fever.
• Perioral Cyanosis + ends.

→ score of severity : *See Mémo 1*

III ♦ Supported in préhospitalier
• Assess.
• Position of comfort.
• O2 if needed for SpO2 ≥ 94%.
• Monitoring (FR, FC, SpO2, NIBP, draw).
• Measurement of the blood glucose levels.
• Measurement of the temperature.
• Track IV rarely necessary
• Reassess regularly.

IV ♦ Processing

• Without sign of severity: Corticosteroids per os.
- Betamethasone 0.05% Po: 20 drops/kg or 0.25 mg/kg
Or
- Prednisolone PO : 1 to 2 mg/kg.
• Moderate laryngitis: Corticosteroids per os +/- aerosol of adrenaline 5 mg, monitoring SAU.
• Severe laryngitis: O2, aerosol of adrenaline 5 mg, corticosteroids per os, Sau Monitoring or Surveillance USC if symptoms remain severe despite the treatment, or if a high number of inhaled treatments is necessary.
• If Track PO not tolerated: methylprednisolone IV: 1 mg/kg.

Think About It

Among the child < 6 months, consider an endoscopic examination ent to eliminate the presence of structural malformation or vascular.

Sub-Part 3
Cardiac pathologies

>>> Mémo 9 - Arrêt cardio-respiratoire

>>> Mémo 10 - Coarctation de l'aorte

>>> Mémo 11 - Infection materno-fœtale

>>> Mémo 12 - Malaise de la tétralogie de Fallot

>>> Mémo 13 - Myocardite

>>> Mémo 14 - Tachycardie supraventriculaire (TSV)

>>> Mémo 15 - Transposition des gros vaisseaux (TGV)

Memo 9

Cardiopulmonary Arrest

I ♦ Definition

The majority of the judgments cardio-respiratory (CAB) are pediatric of origin hypoxic. The asystole is the Pace The most frequent. The prognosis is bleak in case of Paediatric ACR extra-hospital.

Among the child < 1 year, the most frequent cause is the min (see Mémo 32 Mort inattendue du nourrisson).

II ♦ Signs

- AVPU.

Has Alert

V   Response to the voice (voice)

P   Response to pain (bread)

U   No response (unresponsive)

- Apnea or gasping.
- Lack of movement: Absence of pulse, blood pressure.
- Pallor or cyanosis deep.
- Hypoxia-hypercapnia → respiratory arrest → bradycardia → Cardiac arrest/asystole.
- Note the time of no flow and low flow : the prognosis depends on it.
- Assess the Responsiveness of the wards.

III ♦ Supported in préhospitalier

- Unconscious → Yes.
- Call for help, while remaining at the bedside of the child. If two rescuers present: one begins the resuscitation and the other called the relief.

• Open the airway.
• Is this that the breathing is normal? (Look-listen-feel) → not.
• Begin by 5 ventilations (if possible to the Bavu 100% O2): The mask is held with a hand in the form of C (index-inch), the other fingers are positioned in E on the mandible without the compress → signs of life → not.
Insufflation of a duration of one second.
• 15 chest compressions (rhythm 100/120 per minute, although release between compressions). Keep the ratio 15:2, regardless of the number of first-aiders.
• 2 ventilations then 15 chest compressions (if < 1 year • a first-aider: Chest compressions to 2 fingers • two rescuers: compression with inches and the hands around the chest).

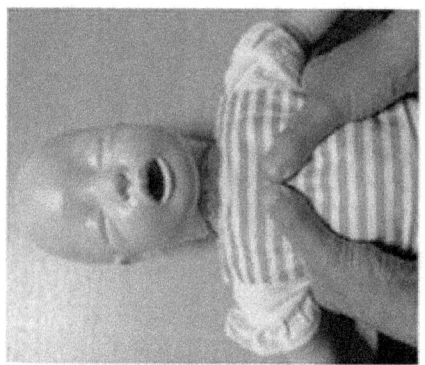
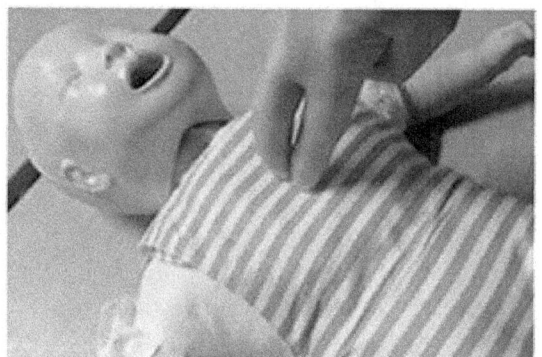

© L./D.
Call the UAS after 1 min of cardio-pulmonary resuscitation if a single first-aider present.

♦ algorithm cardiopulmonary resuscitation
• Installing the scope to assess the Heart Rate: therapeutics in function of the algorithm.
• Install patches to Defib:
- It is possible to use a DSA or DAE from 1 year, with attenuator if available up to 8 years;

- For the infant, manual defibrillator is preferable; however, if not available, the possibility to use the DSA or DAE < 1 year.

>>> **Installing the défébrillateur-position of patches**

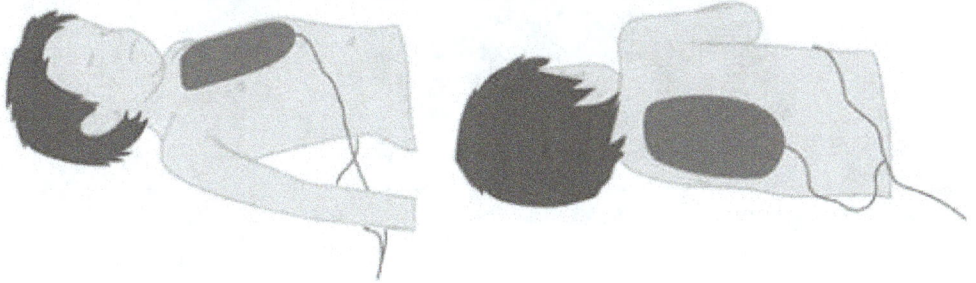

• Intubation and capnography extension.
• Once intubated, cardiac massage (100-120/min)/ventilation (10 breaths/min).
• Tracheal aspiration if needed.
• Obtain a first quick vascular: test VVP < 1 min or IO from the outset.

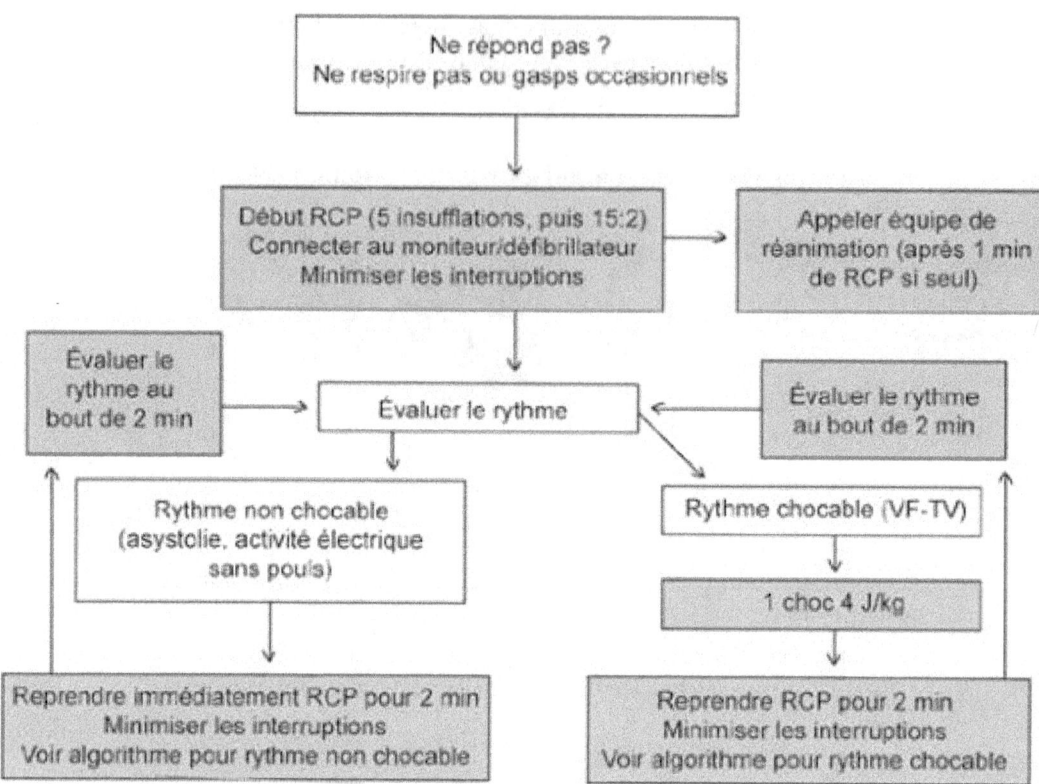

→ If pace not chocable

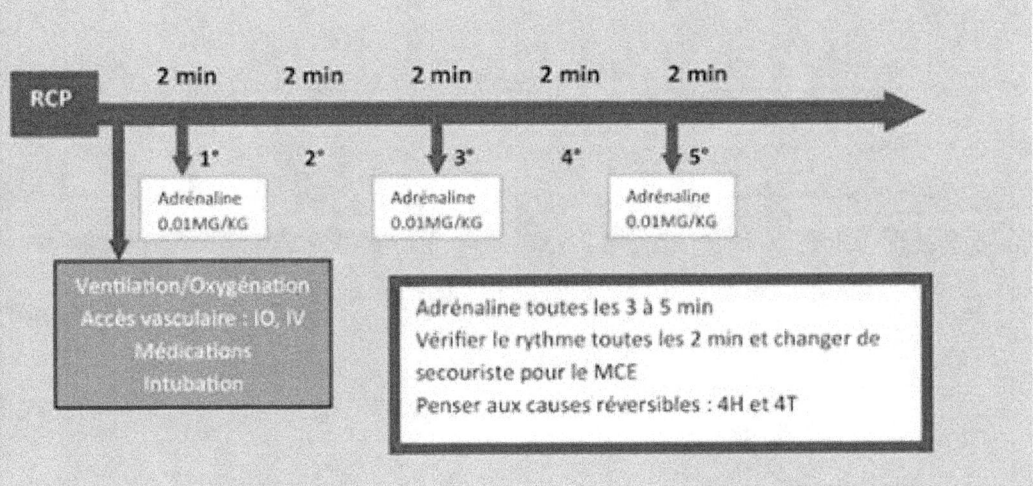

→ If chocable pace

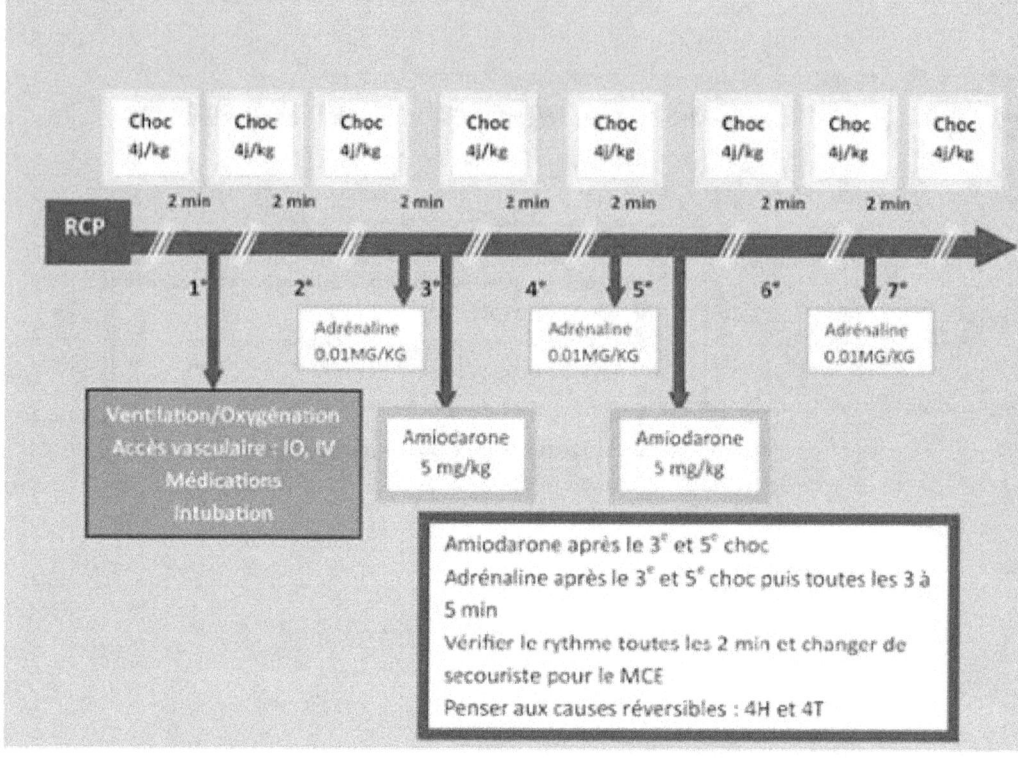

♦ after the beginning of the maneuvers
- Measurement of the rectal temperature.
- Measurement of the blood glucose levels.
- Installing the gastric probe.
- Correct the causes reversible.

4h	4T
Hypoxia	Thrombosis (or Coronary Pulmonary)
Hypovolemia	Tension pneumothorax
Hyper/hypokalemia	Cardiac tamponade

| Hypothermia | Toxic |

IV ♦ Processing

- Adrenaline : dilute 1 mg of adrenaline + 9 ml of NaCl 0.9% and inject in IV = 10 mcg/kg (0.1 ml/kg) all 3-5 minutes.

Attention! The adrenaline is inactivated by the bicarbonate.
- Filling of NaCl 0.9% 20 ml/kg if indicated (→ attention if suspicion of heart failure/myocarditis).
- Bicarbonates (1 mEq/kg) may be considered before a documented acidosis or hyperkalaemia.
- If infectious cause: consider the antibiotic therapy (Cefotaxime 100 mg/kg).
- If atrial fibrillation: shock to 4 joules/kg.

♦ supported post-CSR
- In the case of recovery of a pace, titrate the oxygen in function of the SpO2, adjust the ventilation in function of the pathology and the capnie and PEP in function of the pathology.
- Consider the infusion of adrenaline to maintain the hemodynamic (begin to 0.1 mcg/kg/min).
- Monitor the temperature.
- The child post-judgment must be directed to a paediatric resuscitation.

Think About It

Take into consideration the psychological aspect of the entourage (see Mémo 32 Mort inattendue du nourrisson).

Memo 10
Coarctation of the aorta

I ♦ Definition
Congenital heart disease involving a narrowing more or less severe of the Aortic isthmus. The aortic coarctation can be diagnosed in the antenatal period, postnatal in or among the older child in less severe cases. Among the new-born of a few days, the clinical presentation may mimic a sepsis, and occurs after the closure of the ductus arteriosus. The clinical sign the most important is the difference of palpation between the Pulse Right humeral and femoral Pulse (absent or greatly reduced).

II ♦ Signs

♦ In the newborn up to 3 weeks of life
* Signs of heart failure:
- Difficulty to suck, dyspnoea, diaphoresis;
- Lethargy, vomiting, grayish complexion;
- Hepatomegaly, increase in the work of breathing, crépitants to the lung auscultation;
- Gallop to the cardiac auscultation;
- Systolic murmur among some new-born babies.
* Difference of palpation between the Pulse Right humeral and femoral Pulse (absent or greatly reduced).
* SpO2 Difference between the right hand and the lower limbs.
* Circulatory collapse.

♦ In the child
* Hypertension.
* Decrease in femoral pulse.
* Gradient of blood pressure between the upper and lower limbs.
* Rarely, heart failure left.

III ♦ Supported in préhospitalier

- Monitoring (HR, NBP, SpO2, FR). The saturation should be measured at the level of the right hand and the lower limbs. The PNI must be measured to 4 members.
- Measurement of the blood glucose levels.
- Measurement of the temperature.
- Install VVP → If vascular access difficult, consider installing a KTVO if the cord is still present. Intra-bone in the child greater.
- Extent of lactate if available.
- O2 at need, aim a préductale saturation of approximately 90%. Excessive oxygenation can accelerate the closure of the ductus arteriosus.
- Transfer in emergency on a hospital center benefiting of a service of neonatal resuscitation or pediatric, and ideally a service of paediatric heart surgery.

IV ♦ Processing
- In the new-born: start an infusion of prostaglandin E1. Ideally, the prostaglandins E1 should be administered in a dedicated way.

→ prostaglandins E1 to begin at 0.01-0.05 mcg/kg/min. To adjust depending on the clinical response. Begin at the higher dose if it is suspected that the ductus arteriosus is closed (circulatory collapse to a few days of life, absence of femoral pulse).

→ If possible, consult the Center receiver to discuss the beginning of a treatment by prostaglandins if the status of the child the permits.
- The administration of prostaglandins E1 May cause apneas (increase of the risk in the function of the dose), hypoglycaemia, hypotension, irritability, a flushing, a discomfort or fever.
- Intubation is recommended for cases with a presentation severe (respiratory insufficiency, respiratory collapse) or apneas repeated after the start of infusion of prostaglandins.
- If a is inotropic required, the adrenaline can be started at a low dose (0.1 mcg/kg/min).
- Since in préhospitalier, the final diagnosis may not be confirmed and that the hypothesis of sepsis cannot be excluded, a IV antibiotic therapy should be started (see Mémo 11 Infection materno-foetale).

Think About It

Only the prostaglandins of type PGE1 must be administered in the event of suspicion of cardiac malformation ducto-dependent. Not to be confused with other types of prostaglandins.

Memo 11
Infection maternal-fetal

I ♦ Definition
The infection materno-fetal (IMF) is an infection transmitted in ante-partum or in per-partum of the mother to the child. The Germs are the most common group B streptococci and E. coli. The infections to Listeria are rare but extremely severe. The signs of MFIS are subtle and little specific, it is important to demonstrate a high level of suspicion. Each year, they are responsible for 1 000 to 3 000 sepsis, and 100 to 300 deaths (10 per cent of mortality if the infection is proven, and 10 to 30 per cent of sequelae, including to the Neurological level). They can occur in the absence of risk factors (approximately 5 per cent of the cases).

II ♦ Signs

♦ Risk Factors
• Maternal History: MFIS strepto B during previous pregnancy, hospitalization and prolonged antibiotic therapy during pregnancy.
• Vaginal Levy (PV) positive.
• Maternal ECBU positive.
• Opening Duration of the egg (≥ 18 h).
• Maternal fever ≥ 38 °C (during childbirth and the 2 hours post-childbirth).
• Prematurity unexplained (≤ 36 sa) or premature rupture of the Membranes < 37 SA).
• Jumeau infected.
• Table of chorioamnionitis.
• Tinted Liquid or méconial.
• Perinatal Asphyxia unexplained.

♦ Clinical Signs
• Evoke MFIS in any new-born unstable.
• Respiratory distress, sometimes only isolated geignement (considered as a FMF until proof to the contrary).

* Hemodynamic instability: gray complexion, prolongation of the time of capillary recoloration, tachycardia. The arterial hypotension is a late sign.
* Fever: Rarely present.
* Neurological Impairment: hypotonia, alteration of the state of consciousness, convulsions.
* Achievement of the skin: rash.

III ♦ Supported in préhospitalier
* Monitoring (HR, NBP, SpO2, FR).
* Measurement of the blood glucose levels.
* Measure the temperature.
* Administration O2 → if necessary.
* Install VVP. If vascular access difficult → consider installing a KTVO in the newborn.
* Levies devices and stomach, and hemoculture pre-antibiotic → if possible. Do not delay the antibiotics if not achievable.
* Transfer in resuscitation pediatric or in the intensive care unit as a function of the severity of the clinical signs.

IV ♦ Processing
* Begin a Antibiotic therapy: association of two antibiotics (beta-lactam and aminoglycoside).
- Amoxicillin 50 mg/kg/dose (meningeal dose = 100 mg/kg/dose)
- Gentamicin :

Post Age-conceptionnel	< 30 SA	30-33 its	34-36 its	≥ 37 its
	7 mg/kg	6.5 mg/kg	6 mg/kg	5.5 mg/kg

- Addition of cefotaxime 50 mg/kg/dose (meningeal dose = 100 mg/kg/dose) in severe cases, or in the case of vaginal levy positive for E. coli.

The standard antibiotic therapy for the infection maternal-fetal can vary in function of the practices and the local epidemiology. Check with the regional hospital center of reference in neonatology.

• Ventilatory support according to the clinical condition (NIV or intubation and mechanical ventilation).
• Hemodynamic support if necessary. The noradrenaline is the inotropic choice in cases of sepsis. The initial dose is 0.1 mcg/kg/min and can be titrated depending on the clinical response. During the first day of life, aim an average blood pressure at least equivalent to the number of weeks of amenorrhea.

Think About It

The infection maternal-fetal must always be mentioned in a newborn unstable.

Memo 12

Malaise of the tetralogy of Fallot

I ♦ Definition
The ᵗᵉᵗʳᵃˡᵒᵍʸ ᵒᶠ ᶠᵃˡˡᵒᵗ is a cyanotic congenital heart disease. It can be diagnosed in prenatal or postnatal period. It combines an interventricular septal defect, a pulmonary stenosis, a dextroposition with dilatation of the aorta and a right ventricular hypertrophy.

II ♦ Signs
The malaise of the tetralogy of Fallot is an emergency.
It has for main circumstances déclenchantes:
- The fever;
- The pain;
- The dehydration.

♦ 1st phase: "tonic"

• Restlessness.

• Crying.
• Accentuation of the cyanosis.

• Tachycardia.

♦ 2e phase:"" hypotonic
• Gray complexion and pallor.

• Shallow breathing.

• Tachycardia greater than 140/min.

• Disappearance of the breath to the auscultation of the heart.

• Decline of the vigilance.

• Geignement.

III ♦ Supported in préhospitalier
* Calm the child and avoid the crying.
* Put the child in a position of " squatting " (fetal position, legs folded on the abdomen).

- Measurement of the temperature.
- Measurement of the blood glucose levels.
- Monitoring (cf, FR, SpO2, NBP).
- Install VVP.

IV ♦ Processing
- Diazepam in intrarectal (0.5 mg/kg, max. : 10 mg).
- Propranolol (1 ampoule: 5 ml = 5 mg): dilute 1 ml = 1 mg of propranolol in 4 ml G5%. Inject a first dose of 1 mg IVL, if absence of effectiveness renew the dose.
- Provide an infusion of maintenance COMPENSAL type® G5% and possibly a filling by of macromolecules.
- Take contact with the Cardiology Service where the child is followed. The malaise is an indication to stay ahead of the surgical management of the child.

Think About It

Monitor the capillary blood glucose after injection of propranolol every 6 hours for 24 hours, or more frequently in young infants.

Memo 13
Myocarditis

I ♦ Definition
The ᵐʸᵒᶜᵃʳᵈⁱᵗⁱˢ is a inflammatory pathology of the Myocardium inducing a ventricular dysfunction. It is most often caused by a virus (Enterovirus, influenza, etc.) and may occur as a fulminant or present themselves in a way more frustrates. It is the main cause of heart failure in children with no history. The children achieved are at risk of cardiopulmonary arrest.

II ♦ Signs

♦ flu syndrome
* Headache.
* Asthenia.
* Sore throat.
* Fever.
* Arthralgia.
* Diarrhea.

♦ Cardiac symptoms
* Tachypnea (wheezing, signs of PAO, draw).
* Reduced tolerance to the effort.
* Vomiting, Abdominal pain.
* Difficulty of power (to look especially in the newborn and the smallest infant).
* Chest pain atypical.
* Tachycardia.
* Signs of vasoconstriction: mottled, cold extremities, TRC lying, Pulse Devices evil/not collected.
* Signs of low-flow: oligo-anuria, disorders of the conscience.
* Hepatomegaly, hépatalgie, Hepatojugular reflux, turgor chin strap.

♦ sign of seriousness

• Hypotension.
III ♦ Supported in préhospitalier
• O2 if needed for SpO2 ≥ 94%.
• Monitoring (FR, FC, SpO2, NBP).
• Measurement of the blood glucose, troponin (if possible).
• Measurement of the temperature.
• ECG: ventricular tachycardia, sinus tachycardia, AV block, sus-offset ST, ↑QT, etc.
• Install VVP.
• Reassess regularly.
• Monitoring of the diuresis.
• If available echo: VG dilated and/or hypokinétique.
• Rapid transfer to a hospital center benefiting of a paediatric resuscitation.
→ consider the transfer in a CSR with ECMO (extracorporeal membrane oxygenation), if in the vicinity.

IV ♦ Processing
1) attention to the circulatory filling → may be poorly tolerated.
2) for inotropic support the Myocardium: dobutamine, adrenaline.
3) Diuretic: furosemide 1 mg/kg.
4) Disorder of the pace possible.
5) In the case of increasing requirements in O2, A NIV can be attempted. Intubation should preferably be done in specialized center because the risk of SCA is important.
6) corticosteroids and immunoglobulins.
7) ECMO if failure, severe.

Think About It

The clinical presentation in the infant may look like a bronchiolitis.

Memo 14
Supraventricular tachycardia (SVT)

I ♦ Definition
The ^{SVT} is the arrhythmia the more common among the child. More commonly, the ^{tachycardia} is to QRS purposes, the P wave is visible in 60% of cases, and the heart rhythm is regular.

II ♦ Signs
* Heart rate > 200 in the newborn and > 180 among the child.
* Asthenia.
* Signs of circulatory insufficiency: mottles, hepatomegaly, cold extremities.
* Vomiting.
* Food difficulties.
* May be associated with fever, a virus or a myocarditis.

III ♦ Supported in préhospitalier
* Monitoring (cf, FR, SpO2, NBP).
* ECG.
* Measurement of the temperature.
* Measurement of the blood glucose levels.
* Reduction by vagal maneuvers:

- In the infant:
- Pocket of ice on the face for a few seconds in order to generate an effect of surprise, to maintain 2-3 seconds (10 s in total) after reduction;
- Installation of gastric probe or probe of aspiration.

- Among the grand child:
- Carotid massage;
- The compressions ocular (as Valsalva maneuver) likely to cause sequelae, they are no longer practiced.
* Install VVP if needed.

IV ♦ Processing

• If ineffectiveness of vagal maneuvers:

- STRIADYNE® 1 mg/kg (max. dose Of 10 mg for the first dose, 20 mg max. for subsequent doses);

Or

Adenosine - 0.1 mg/kg max. 6 mg, then 0.2 mg/kg, max. 12 mg for other injections.

Inject in flash in the fold of the left elbow to the more close to the heart if possible (very short half-life). During the injection, a ECG trace is achieved, noted above the time of the injection.

The injection of these treatments gives the child a sensation of unease intense. It causes bradycardia at the time of the action of the STRIADYNE®. Prepare the atropine 20 mcg/kg and administer the need.

To make available the resuscitation equipment.

• If failure of other therapeutic or serious instability at the outset: synchronous cardioversion: 1 Impact = 1 Joule/kg, then 2 joules/kg.

• Transfer to a hospital center with a cardiopédiatre on the structure if possible.

Think About It

Attention! The STRIADYNE® and the adenosine may cause a bronchospasm in patients with asthma.

Memo 15

Transposition of the great vessels (TGV)

I ♦ Definition
Congenital heart disease involving an inversion of the implementation of the large vessels. As well the aorta takes birth at the level of the right ventricle and the pulmonary artery to the level of the left ventricle. The TGV is more and more often diagnosed in the antenatal period, but is also sometimes diagnosed in postnatal. The clinical presentation can be extremely severe as soon the birth if the septum is intact.

II ♦ Signs
* Cyanosis refractory to the oxygen.
* Little or no respiratory distress.
* Femoral Pulse present (in opposition to the coarctation of the aorta).
* Heart murmur little or not present.
* Differential of saturation pre (right hand) and post-ductale (lower limbs).
* Circulatory collapse fast in cases where the foramen ovale is little permeable.

III ♦ Supported in préhospitalier
* Monitoring (HR, NBP, SpO2, FR). The saturation should be measured at the level of the right hand and the lower limbs. The PNI must be measured to 4 members.
* Measurement of the blood glucose levels.
* Measure the temperature.
* Install VVP. If vascular access difficult, consider installing a KTVO in the newborn.
* Extent of lactate if available.
* Transfer in emergency on a hospital center benefiting of a service of neonatal resuscitation or pediatric, and ideally a service of paediatric heart surgery. The new-born with TGV may require a

atrioseptostomie of emergency (procedure of Rashkind). The transport to a specialized center must be rapid.

IV ♦ Processing

*After discussion with the Center receiver, start an infusion of prostaglandin E1.
- Ideally, prostaglandins E1 should be administered in a dedicated way.
- Prostaglandins E1 to begin at 0.01-0.05 mcg/kg/min. To adjust depending on the clinical response. If possible, consult the Center receiver to discuss the beginning of a treatment by prostaglandins if the status of the child the permits.
- The administration of PGE1 may cause apneas, hypoglycaemia, hypotension, irritability, a flushing, discomfort or fever.
- If possible and safe, the child should be transferred in spontaneous ventilation. Intubation is recommended only for patients with a severe Presentation (metabolic acidosis severe, collapse) or of repeated apneas result at the beginning of the infusion of prostaglandins.
- If a is inotropic required, the adrenaline can be started at a low dose (0.1 mcg/kg/min).
*Since in préhospitalier, the final diagnosis may not be confirmed and that the hypothesis of sepsis cannot be excluded, a IV antibiotic therapy should be started (see Mémo 11 Infection materno-fœtale).

Think About It

The clinical presentation of a TGV non-diagnosed in antenatal can mimic a PAH neonatal. Think about when a new-born remains cyanotic despite a supported optimized.

Sub-Part 4
Neurological pathologies

>>> Mémo 16 - Crise convulsive

>>> Mémo 17 - Encéphalite

>>> Mémo 18 - État de mal convulsif

>>> Mémo 19 - Hypertension intracrânienne (HTIC)

>>> Mémo 20 - Méningite

Memo 16

Convulsive crisis

I ♦ Definition
Electrical Discharge of the paroxysmal cerebral cortex. The causes can be multiple. Although frequent, the febrile seizures are straightforward and are a diagnosis of elimination.

II ♦ Signs
• Muscular contractures tonic and/or generalized clonic or a portion isolated from the body.
• Convulsions may present themselves in a more subtle way by pupil abnormalities, mâchonnements, blinks the eyes, loss of tone, etc.
• Loss of knowledge.
• Loss of urine.
• Bites of language.
• Tachycardia, hypertension.
• Noisy breathing and jerky.
• Fever.

♦ signs of seriousness
• Duration and frequency of crises.
• Duration of phase post-critical.
• State of convulsive evil if prolonged crisis and/or repeated for more than 20 minutes (see Mémo 18 État de mal convulsif).
• Cyanosis, breaks or apneas.

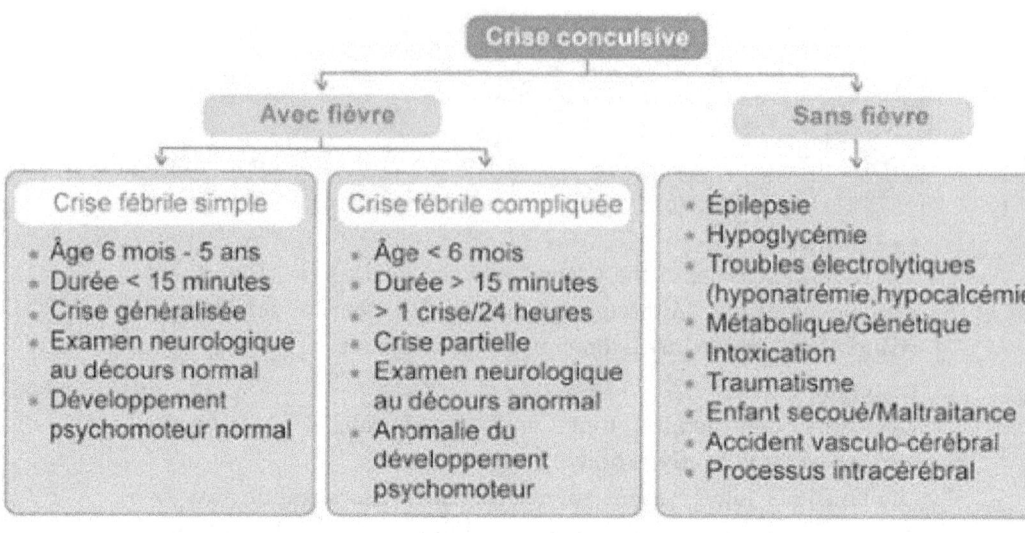

III ♦ Supported in préhospitalier
* Put in lateral position of security.
* Release of the airway.
* O2 at MHC if persistent cyanosis or to maintain a SpO2 > 94%.
* Monitoring (cf, FR, SpO2, NBP).
* Measurement of the blood glucose levels.
* Measurement of the temperature.
* Install VVP if necessary.
* Examination:
- Description of the crisis;
- Duration of the crisis+++;
- If repeated crises, neurological condition and awakening between the crises;
- Signs associated: trauma, HTA known, intoxication, metabolic disease, etc.;
- Infectious symptoms Concomitant: vomiting, diarrhea, respiratory symptoms, general state pre-crisis, skin rash, etc.;
- Personal ATCD (psychomotor development) and family.
* Clinical Examination complete neurological.

IV ♦ Processing

→ If fever, administer an antipyretic in function of the last dose received (see Mémo 29 Fièvre).
→ If phase post-critical = clinical examination and monitoring.
→ If the convulsion is of a duration of more than 5 min, Administer diazepam intra-rectal (IR) or midazolam intra-jugal (IJ). If the convulsion persists for more than 5 min after the dose of benzodiazepine IR or Ij, a maintenance dose of benzodiazepine IV, such clonazepam IV, must be administered. If the crisis does not yield → **see** Mémo 18 État de mal convulsif.

Medicine	Posology	Repetition	Maximum	Precautions
Midazolam	0.3 mg/kg in intra-jugal, Or for the BUCCOLAM® : - 2.5 mg < 1 year - 5 mg between 1 and 5 years - 7.5 mg between 5 and 10 years - 10 mg >10 years		10 mg/dose	If volume of more than 1 ml, separate the dose between the two cheeks
Diazepam	0.5 mg/kg IR	The injection may be	10 mg/dose	Do not dilute

		repeated 10 to 20 minutes after		
Clonazepam	0.05 - 0.1 mg/kg IV	0.1 mg/kg/6 h	1 mg/dose	Administer on 2 min

Think About It

The blood glucose must be quickly measured for all children who convulsent or in a state post-critical. In the case of hypoglycaemia: G10% 2 ml/kg if < 5 kg or g30% 1 ml/kg IVD if > 5 kg (may be given on a track device) or glucagon IM 1 mg.

And then begin a continuous infusion of polyionique G10%.

Check glucose 15 minutes after the injection.

Memo 17
Encephalitis

I ♦ Definition
Pathology febrile acute whose symptoms evoke an infringement of the central nervous system.

II ♦ Signs
* Fever.
* Alteration of the conscience.
* Disorder of the behavior.
* Partial crises or generalized.
* Motor Deficit localized.
* Signs of increased intracranial pressure:
- Eyes in sunset;
- Headache;
- Mushroom Fontanelle;
- Vomiting;
- Triad of Cushing (bradycardia, HTA, irregularity of the respiratory rhythm).

III ♦ Supported in préhospitalier
* Examination:
- Description of the crisis or crises if there is place;
- If repeated crises, neurological condition and awakening between the crises;
- Infectious symptoms Concomitant: vomiting, diarrhea, respiratory symptoms, general state pre-crisis, skin rash, etc.;
- Personal ATCD (psychomotor development) family and;
- Clinical examination complete neurological.
* Release of the airway (PLS if disorder of the conscience).
* O2 at MHC if persistent cyanosis or to maintain a SpO2 > 94%.
* Monitoring (cf, FR, SpO2, NBP).
* Measurement of the blood glucose levels.
* Measurement of the temperature.
* Install VVP.

IV ♦ Processing
Aciclovir : 20 mg/kg/8 h or 500 mg/m2/8 H in IV during 21 days.
• The neurological condition may require intubation if the patient does not protects more its respiratory tract.
• Transfer in emergency on a hospital center benefiting of a resuscitation service pediatric.

Think About It

Any table of acute encephalitis with disorder of the febrile conscience is a herpes encephalitis until proof to the contrary.

Memo 18
State of convulsive incorrectly

I ♦ Definition
Succession of seizures without recovery of consciousness between them or when a seizure activity continues to extend beyond 20 minutes.

II ♦ Signs
* Muscular contractures tonic and/or generalized clonic or an isolated part of the body.
* Convulsions may present themselves in a more subtle way by pupil abnormalities, mâchonnements, blinks the eyes, loss of tone, etc.
* Loss of knowledge.
* Tachycardia, hypertension.
* Noisy breathing and jerky.
* Persistence of these signs without recovery of consciousness post-critical > 20 min.

III ♦ Supported Pre-hospital
* Ensure the release of the airway (cannula of Guédel, PLS).
* Monitoring (cf, FR, SpO2, NBP).
* Oxygen therapy to the MHC.
* Measurement of the blood glucose levels.
* Measurement of the temperature.
* Install VVP.

Think About It

• Patients with Epilepsy complex have often a treatment plan in the event of a crisis, developed by their physician. Make the request to the parents.

* Always eliminate the presence of a hypoglycaemia (see Mémo 16 Crise convulsive).

IV ♦ Processing

```
┌─────────────────────────────────┐
│     Traitement de 1re ligne     │
│         Benzodiazépine          │
│  CI : Syndrome de Lennox-Gastaut│
└─────────────────────────────────┘
```

Si pas de voie IV :
Diazépam 0,5 mg/kg IR
(max 10 mg/dose)
Ou **Midazolam intra jugal**
0,3 mg/kg (max 10mg/dose)

Si voie IV :
Clonazepam 0,05 mg/kg IVL
(dose max 1 mg/dose)
Si deuxième dose :
0,1 mg/kg IVL sur 6 h.

Ou **Lorazepam** 0,1 mg/kg IVL
(max 4 mg/dose)

Si échec après 5 minutes
Répéter une deuxième dose de benzodiazépine.
Favoriser dose IV/IO

Si échec
Traitement de 2e ligne

Phénytoïne
15 mg/kg IVL sur 20 min, dans serum physiologique seul,
bien rincer car peut boucher les KT et IO (max 1000 mg/dose).

Après 30 minutes

Phénobarbital
Nné : 20 mg/kg
Enfant : 15 mg/kg
IVL sur 20 min
(max 600 mg/dose)
(CI :syndrome de Dravet)

- Intubation : doit être envisagée à tout moment si arrêt respiratoire ou désaturation malgré apport O₂.
- La majorité des états de mal convulsif n'aura pas besoin d'être intubé.
- Si intubation :
ISR avec propofol.
Éviter le NESDONAL®.
Éviter curare longue action car peut camoufler l'activité convulsive.

Si échec
Traitement de 3e ligne
(nécessite le plus souvent intubation et ventilation mécanique).
Patient devra être mis sous EEG continu en réanimation pédiatrique.

Nouveaux traitements en émergence :
- Levetiracetam IV.
- Valproate de sodium
Après discussion avec l'équipe de neurologie, ou chez un patient épileptique avec protocole de soins.

BZD en perfusion continue : **Midazolam IV**
200 à 500 mcg /kg IVD.
Puis 2 mcg/kg/min (=120 mcg/kg/h).
Doubler la dose/15 min
+ répéter bolus150 mcg/kg toutes les 30 min.
Max : 20 mcg/kg/min (= 1 200 mcg/kg/h)

Barbituriques : **Thiopenthal IV**
5 mg/kg IVL sur 1 heure.
Puis 0,5 à 5 mg/kg/h.
Attention : hypotension artérielle fréquente.
Peut nécessiter remplissage et amines.

Memo 19
Intracranial hypertension (HTIC)

I ♦ Definition
Abnormal rise in the intracranial pressure. Among the child, can be caused in particular by: head trauma, brain tumor, meningitis, hydrocephalus, intracranial hematoma, thrombosis.

II ♦ Signs
* Eyes in sunset.
* Headache.
* Fontanel convex.
* Vomiting (particularly early risers) and/or difficulty to the power supply.
* Triad of Cushing (bradycardia, HTA, irregularity of the respiratory rhythm).
* Behavior Disorders.
* Pupillary asymmetry.
* Strabismus.
* Hypotonia.
* Seizure.
* In infants, the possibility of an increase in the cranial perimeter (refer to the book of health).

III ♦ Supported in préhospitalier
* Monitoring (cf, FR, SpO2, NBP).
* Measurement of the blood glucose levels.
* Measurement of the temperature.
* O2 if necessary.
* Install VVP.
* Aim for a normoglycémie, normocapnie (35-40 mmHg), normothermic, avoid hypotension (AIM PAM > 55 If 2 years and less, and > 65 If 2-10 years), and desaturation.
* Position the child head straight to foster the venous drainage, elevated to 30o.

IV ♦ Processing
* Intubation in rapid sequence according to the clinical condition (ketamine 3-4 mg/kg if < 2 years, or etomidate 0.2-0.4 mg/kg if 2 years and more, in association with succinylcholine 2 mg/kg if < 18 months, or 1 mg/kg if > 18 months). Monitoring Post-intubation of expired CO_2.
* Salted Serum hypertonic 7.5% : 3-6 ml/kg in 15-20 min.
* Mannitol 20%: 0.5 g/kg in 10-15 min.
* Ensure sedation-adequate analgesia.
* Corticosteroids in the event of a brain tumor, to discuss with the service receiver.

Think About It

The shaken baby syndrome (violent shaking inflicted on the child), form the more lethal abuse, can cause of intracranial injury with signs of HTIC: reporting is done in a second time by the hospital service before the results of examinations.

Memo 20
Meningitis

I ♦ Definition
Infection of the meninges of origin viral or bacterial.

II ♦ Signs
* Headache.
* Vomiting and/or refusal of food.
* Phono and photophobia.
* Fever (high and abrupt onset).
* Stiffness of the neck.
* Kernig's sign (lower member in bending at the level of the knee and the hip, pain or resistance when the extension of the lower member at the level of the knee).
* Signs of Brudzinski (flexion reflex of the thighs during the deflection of the neck).
* Behavior Disorders.
* Hyperesthesia skin.
* In infants < 18 months:
- Overall hypotonia;
- Fontanel tense (sitting, without tears).

♦ signs of seriousness
* Disorders of the conscience.
* Neurological signs of focus.
* Convulsions.
* Purpura.
* Hemodynamic disorders.

III ♦ Supported in préhospitalier
* Port of a mask by the staff and the close entourage.
* Monitoring (HR, NBP, SpO2, FR).
* Measurement of the blood glucose levels.
* Measure the temperature.

* Examination:
- Start and importance of signs;
- Concept of contage;
- State of vaccinations.
* Install VVP.
* Under O2 if necessary.
* Transfer in emergency on a hospital center benefiting of a resuscitation service pediatric.

IV ♦ Processing
* If hemodynamic disorders → vascular filling 20 ml/kg of physiological serum on 20 min to renew if necessary.
* Urgent Antibiotic therapy:
- Ceftriaxone 100 mg/kg/dose, or cefotaxime 200 to 300 mg/kg in 4 times (depends of the bacterium);
- Amoxicillin : 200 to 300 mg/kg/24 h in the case of suspicion of Listeria;
- Associated with gentamicin 5 mg/kg if less than 3 months (E. coli)
* Treatment antipyretic and analgesic: paracetamol (15 mg/kg every 6 h).
* Support for convulsions according to the usual treatments (see Mémo 16 Crise convulsive and Mémo 18 État de mal convulsif).
* If suspicion of bacterial meningitis, consider dexamethasone 0.15 mg/kg.
* The neurological condition may require intubation if the patient does not protects more its respiratory tract.

Think About It

Take knowledge of the Vaccination book of the child, however there are rare cases of meningitis pneumococcal despite vaccination.

To consider if suspicion of pneumococcus resistant (rare in France)

→ vancomycin 15 mg/kg/dose (60 mg/kg/24 h) or by continuous infusion.

Sub-Part 5
Traumatology

>>> Mémo 21 - Polytraumatisé

Memo 21
With multisystem trauma

I ♦ Definition

Injuries are the leading cause of death for children over 1 year in France. More than 80 per cent of children polytraumatisés have a head trauma associated.

Falls and accidents of the public road are the causes of the most frequent traumas among children. The penetrating trauma is rare in pediatrics.

The kinetics of the accident allows to anticipate the severity and type of lesions.

II ♦ Signs

♦ respiratory signs
- Signs of a struggle.
- Cyanosis.
- Auscultation asymmetric.
  Rapid shallow breathing •/bradypnée or apnea.
- Subcutaneous emphysema.
- Desaturation.

♦ circulatory Signs
- Tachycardia.
- Hypotension (may be late, associated with a poor prognosis).
- Time of dermal recoloration > 3 seconds.
- Cold extremities, mottles.
- Alteration of the state of consciousness.
- Massive hemorrhage extériorisée.
- Abdomen painful.

♦ neurological signs
- Alteration of the state of consciousness:
  - AVPU

A = alert
V = response to the voice (voice)
P = response to pain (bread)
U = No response (unresponsive)
- Pediatric Glasgow: see Mémo 1.
* Signs of HTIC:
- Pupillary asymmetry;
- Triad of Cushing (bradycardia, HTA, irregularity of the respiratory rhythm).
* Headache, persistent vomiting.
* Convulsions.

III ♦ Supported in préhospitalier

♦ Objectives of the supported
- Recognize and deal with the vital distress cases.
- Prevent the lethal triad (acidosis, coagulopathy, hypothermia).
- Prevent ACSOS (assaults Secondary brain of systemic Origin: Hypotension, hypoxia, hypo or hypercapnia, anemia).
* Monitoring (cf, FR, SpO2, NBP).
* Immobilization of the vertebral column (installation of cervical collar, precaution of hitch).

♦ taken in respiratory load
* Opening of the airway.
* O2 at MHC.
* Aspirations of secretion to the need.
* Thoracic decompression: exsufflation to needle (catheter 18 g) or install thoracic drain if suspicion Pneumothorax Hemothorax/.
* Consider the orotrachea (not of intubation nasotrachéale) if severe respiratory distress despite the initial support, Glasgow ≤ 8.

Induction in rapid sequence:
* < 2 years:
- Ketamine 3-4 mg/kg;
- Suxaméthonium : 2 mg/kg.
* > 2 years:
- Etomidate 0.2-0.4 mg/kg;
- Suxaméthonium : 1 mg/kg.

Sedation relay post-intubation:
- Midazolam 100 mcg/kg/h;
- Sufentanil 0.3 mcg/kg/h.

Post-intubation:
- Installation of probe oro-gastric post-intubation;
- Aim at a expired CO2 between 35-40 mmHg.

♦ **Supported circulatory**
The hemorrhage is the first cause of shock to the with multisystem trauma.
* Install VVP (if possible 2 catheters large caliber) if failure install intra-bone.
= solute without glucose (saline) except if hypoglycaemia.
* Control of bleeding:
- Externalised: Installation of tourniquets, hemostatic dressings, bandages compression bandages;
- Immobilization fracture of the pelvis, traction, femur fracture.
* Make a HémoCue®.
* Circulatory Filling: 20 ml/kg of physiological saline. After 30-40ml/kg inotropic consider (noradrenaline: begin to 0.1 mcg/kg/min) and globular pellet if available.
* Objectives of blood pressure:

	≤ 2 years	2 to 10 years
NEUROTRAUMA	PAM ≥ 55 mm Hg	PAM ≥ 65 mm Hg
ABSENCE OF neurotrauma	PAM ≥ 45 mm Hg	PAM ≥ 55 mm Hg

Proposed by G. Orliaguet-Necker adapted from Haque MCCPS 2007
* If hemodynamic instability or massive bleeding, administration of tranexamic acid: 10-15 mg/kg on 10 min (max. : 1 g).

♦ **Supported neurological**

* Aim for a normoglycémie, normocapnie, normothermic, avoid hypotension, and desaturation.
* Avoid the compression of the jugular veins with the cervical collar (decrease of the venous drainage of the brain).
* In the case of thrust of HTIC:
- Serum hypertonic salted 7.5% : 3 ml/kg;
- Mannitol 20%: 0.5 g/kg;
- Adequate analgesia.

♦ Other
* Measuring the temperature and prevention of hypothermia.
* Measurement of the blood glucose levels.
* Perform a full clinical examination in search of lesions associated.
* If available ultrasound: Fast Echo and search of pneumothorax.
* Immobilization of members if suspicion of fractures.
* Antibiotic therapy if open fracture: clavulanic acid + amoxicillin 50 mg/kg.
* Analgesia in the patient non-intubated:
- Paracetamol : 15 mg/kg in IV;
- Morphine : dose of load: 50 to 100 mcg/kg then 25 mcg/kg in titration.

♦ Orientation
The with multisystem trauma requires a transport to a center of pediatric trauma (if possible) after an evaluation and a initial support fast.

Think About It

Child abuse is a cause of multiple trauma in the child.

Sub-Part   **6**
Other

>>> Mémo 22 - Accouchement à domicile

>>> Mémo 23 - Acidocétose diabétique

>>> Mémo 24 - Anaphylaxie

>>> Mémo 25 - Brûlure

>>> Mémo 26 - Choc septique/Purpura fulminans

>>> Mémo 27 - Diarrhée et déshydratation

>>> Mémo 28 - Électrisé

>>> Mémo 29 - Fièvre

>>> Mémo 30 - Intoxications

>>> Mémo 31 - Malaise du nourrisson

>>> Mémo 32 - Mort inattendue du nourrisson (MIN)

>>> Mémo 33 - Noyade

>>> Mémo 34 - Réanimation du nouveau-né

Memo 22
Home Birth

I ♦ Definition
Home to a new-born born in non-hospital settings.
Rapid assessment of the situation: the end of the pregnancy, twins or not, follow-up of the pregnancy, antenatal diagnosis of congenital pathology, delay of growth in-utero, gestational diabetes, infectious risk. This rapid assessment will quickly request for reinforcements: Paediatric EMS if distress of the new-born, prematurity.

II ♦ signs of a good adaptation to extrauterine life
• Cris/crying.
• Ventilation effective and autonomous.
• Pink complexion.

III ♦ Supported in préhospitalier
• If possible, prepare in upstream of the equipment for the home of the new-born:
- Towel or Lange to lengthen the new-born;
- Clamps of Barr + Kocher clamps + pairs of sterile scissors or scalpel;
- Sterile gloves;
- Compresses + antiseptic;
- Aspirator + probes;
- Equipment for drying the new-born (bonnet, towels, polyethylene bag);
- Scope;
- Prepare near the resuscitation equipment, O2, Bavu, equipment of intubation.
• Note the time of the birth, which will, in a second time, to rate the Apgar: See Mémo 1.
• Prevention of hypothermia: Wrap the new-born in a Lange, the wipe, dry, the styling of a bonnet. Put the child in skin to skin with

her mother to prevent the energy losses (if this is not possible, because of the condition of the mother or the child, put the new-born in a polyethylene bag).
• Monitoring of the temperature at the birth and throughout the supported (target temperature between 36,5o and 37.5o).
• Otherwise transport in normal cell heated++ and by limiting exposure to the cold.
• Clamp the umbilical cord to 10 cm of the umbilicus of the new-born, place another clamp 5 cm further, the section of the cord will be between the two clamps using a sterile scissors or a scalpel.
• The oropharyngeal aspiration is not systematic if the child adapts normally. If necessary, suction brief, oral and nasal (probe no. 8/10, < 150 cm H20).
• Make a blood glucose at birth if neonatal suffering, resuscitation and special risks (maternal diabetes, hypothermia, delayed growth in utero, prematurity): > 2.2 mmol/L (0.6 g/l), variable threshold according to the term, measurement done at the heel, from 15 minutes of life.
If not suffering neonatal, make a blood glucose at 30 minutes of life.
• Monitoring (cf - PNI - SpO2), if poor adaptation or prematurity: See Mémo 1.
• Transportation in the Incubator if new-born hypotherme labile, or ≤ 2500 gr.

IV ♦ Processing
→ If poor adaptation to the extrauterine life, undertake the maneuvers of resuscitation (see Mémo 34 Réanimation du nouveau-né).
→ If hypoglycaemia:
- Implementation within if desire to breast-feeding and in the absence of distress;
- Resucrage per os: 3 ml of G10% to the syringe in the mouth.
→ If failure of the enteral track or if blood glucose levels ≤ 0.6 mmol/l: VVP + G10% 2 ml/kg, and then begin a continuous infusion of polyionique G10% 3 ml/kg/h.
Vitamin K1 per os for the new-born at term: 2 mg/0.2 ml or IV 1 mg.

→ If infectious context, begin the antibiotic therapy (see Mémo 11 Infection materno-fœtale).

♦ Orientation
If good adaptation to the extrauterine life, transfer of the new-born with his mother in the maternity.

Think About It

Establish a birth certificate dated and signed with the exact place of birth.

Memo 23
Diabetic ketoacidosis

I ♦ Definition
The diabetic ketoacidosis is the result of a total deficiency or relative insulin.
Revealing of diabetes in 25 to 30% of cases in the child or complicating a diabetes, known (poor control of the disease, insulin pump and non-compliance with the instructions of monitoring, adolescence).
Among the child, diabetes is essentially type I.
• Hyperglycaemia > 11 mmol/l (2 g/l) and glycosuria ≥ 30 g/L; pH < 7,30 and/or bicarbonate < 15 mmol/L; cétonémie ≥ 0.6 mmol/l or ketones +++.
3 stages followed:
- The ketosis (presence of ketones in the blood and urine);
- The ketoacidosis: ketosis resulting in a decrease in the pH below 7,30 or bicarbonate < 15 mmol/l.
- The coma acidocétosique: ketoacidosis with disorders of the conscience.

II ♦ Signs
• Polyuria, polydipsia from a few weeks to a few months.
• Enuresis.
• Dehydration and weight loss.
• Nausea, vomiting.
• Abdominal pain.
• Shallow breathing.
• Acidosis (acetone odour of the breath).

♦ signs of seriousness
• < 5 years.
• Severe dehydration.
• Disorders of consciousness (Glasgow Coma Score < 12).
• Collapse.

* Respiratory distress.
* Hyperglycaemia > 33.3 mmol/l (6 g/l), pH < 7.10.
* Hypocapnia (PCO2 ≤ 15 mmHg).
* Hypokalemia.

♦ Major complications
* Cerebral edema (more common in children less than 2 years).
* Hypokalemia and disorders of the pace.

III ♦ Supported in préhospitalier
* Monitoring (FR, FC, NBP, SpO2).
* Measure the time of recoloration skin.
* Oxygen therapy if need, aim SpO2 > 94%.
* Compendium of urine (for quantifying the diuresis and iono urinary).
* Measurement of blood glucose monitoring and all 30 minutes for 2 hours and then all the hours for adaptation of the treatment.
* Measurement of the cétonémie (all hours) and/or of the ketones.
* Measurement of the temperature.
* Monitoring the neurological status (Glasgow pediatric).
* Do an ECG, search for signs of hypokalemia.
* Fitting 2 VVP if possible (1 for insulin, 1 for rehydration).
* Blood samples for blood glucose, cétonémie, blood iono, creatinine, osmolarity, calcium, phosphorus, insulin levels.
* Leave the patient in the fasting state during the duration of the treatment IV.
* Note the time of the start of the insulin therapy.

IV ♦ Processing
* In the case of collapse: 1 filling of NaCl 0.9% 20 ml/kg on 20 to 30 min (attention to the risk of cerebral edema especially in infants).
* Take notice with the center of Pediatric Endocrinology referent.

● Insulin

- Rapid-acting insulin (100 IU/ml) get a dilution of 1 ml = 1 IU (well bleed the tubing)
- IVSE insulin

Target: Decrease the blood glucose levels from 2 to 5 mmol/h

Ensure that the corrected kaliéme is ≥ 2 mmol/l otherwise differ the insulin:
→ 0.1 IU/kg/h if pH < 7.20 and age > 5 years and not insulin received in the 8 previous H
→ 0.05 IU/kg/h in all other cases
Adjust the insulin flow to each capillary blood glucose (all 30 minutes of H0 to H2).

< 8.8 mmol/l	Decrease insulin flow of 20%
< 3.3 mmol/l	1 ml/kg of G 30% in SCI + decrease insulin flow of 20%
Decrease > 5.5 mmol/L in 1 h	Decrease insulin flow of 20%

Attention! Do not bolus of insulin! Never stop the insulin even if normalization of the blood glucose, contribution of glucose.
• Simultaneously from H0 to H2 from the outset or after restoration of the blood volume:
- NaCl 0.9% + KCL to 7.46%: 20 ml/l, or 20 mmol/l of K+ added
→ to the flow rate of 8 ml/kg/h if Na corrected < 138 mmol/l or age < 5 years
→ For Speed 10 ml/kg/h in the other cases, do not exceed 500 ml/h
• Contribution of K
If the presence of T waves flattened or K+ corrected < 2 mmol/l and diuresis +: add 20 mmol/l of K to the previous solution and defer the insulin
• To H2, change of infusion on the base 3 l/m2/i according to the ionos and protocol for the service of Pediatric Endocrinology referent
• If signs of HTIC:
- Mannitol 20%: 0.5 g/kg in 10-15 min

- Position the child head straight to foster the venous drainage, elevated to 30°.
* Transfer in paediatric resuscitation:
- Children < 2 years (or even < 5 years)
- If persistent collapse after 20 ml/kg of NaCl 0.9%
- If severe ketoacidosis: pH < 7.10, bicarbonate < 5 mmol/l
- Glasgow Coma Score < 12 or signs of cerebral edema
- Need O2 ≥ 3 l/min, pulmonary edema

For the other, it is desirable to transfer in an emergency service of a hospital with a specialty of endocrino pediatric.

Think About It

* Do not put bicarbonate: risk of cerebral edema.

* Know how to recognize the signs of cerebral edema, rare complication but the prognosis dark (20 to 25 per cent of Death).

* **Calculation of the body surface area in m2 :** $(4 \times \text{weight (kg)} + 7)/(\text{weight (kg)} + 90)$

Calculation corrected serum sodium: Na measured + (blood glucose (mmol/l) - 5)/3

Calculation potassium corrected: Measured K - 6 × (7.40 - pH)

* Namely: blood glucose at 1 g/L = 5.5 mmol/l.

Memo 24
Anaphylaxis

I ♦ Definition
Anaphylaxis is a generalized allergic reaction severe and rapid onset which can cause death. It usually occurs in the minutes or sometimes the hours following exposure to an allergen. Food allergens are the provocative elements the more frequent among children.

II ♦ Signs

♦ **The Anaphylaxis can affect several systems**
* The **Skin** : urticaria, angiedema, pruritus, reached eye (tearing, swelling, redness).
* : Respiratory nasal congestion, sneeze, bronchospasm, upper airway obstruction secondary to the edema (stridor, voice stifled, increase in the work of breathing, dysphagia).
* **Cardiovascular** : state of shock (Tachycardia, hypotension, pulse spinning), possible collapse.
* **Digestive** : vomiting, diarrhea, abdominal pain.
* **Neurological** • : dizziness, alteration of the state of consciousness.

♦ **signs of seriousness**
* A: edema, stridor, hoarseness.
* B: tachypnea, wheezing, fatigue, cyanosis, SpO2 < 92%, confusion.
* C: pallor, vasodilatées ends, TA Low, weakness, coma.

III ♦ Supported in préhospitalier
* Immediately cease the exposure to the allergen if it is still present.
* Monitoring (HR, NBP, SpO2, FR).
* Administration of O2 to need.
* For severe cases, installing a VVP or a track IO. Do not delay the processing by adrenaline IM.
* Any anaphylactic reaction, even if rapid resolution of symptoms after the injection of adrenaline IM (by witnesses or by the emergency services), must be monitored in a hospital because of

the risk of a biphasic reaction. Except in the cases very severe and refractory to treatment, this monitoring can be done in the UAA.

IV ♦ Processing
• Little import the manifestations of anaphylaxis, adrenaline is the treatment of choice. It must be administered quickly. The intramuscular route is the route of choice initially, because it allows a more rapid absorption and plasma levels higher than the subcutaneous injection. The preferred site is the anterolateral aspect of the thigh:
- By auto-injector (ANAPEN®, Epipen®): < 25 kg: 0.15 mg and > 25 kg: 0.3 mg;
- Adrenaline IM (1 mg = 1 ml): 10 mcg/kg/dose (max. dose : 500 mcg);
- The IM dose may be repeated every 5 to 10 min to the need;
- The dose IV or IO of adrenaline must be reserved for the anaphylactic shock refractory to doses IM of adrenaline. It must be administered with caution by an experienced practitioner. The dose is 1 mcg/kg/dose in the child (max. dose : 50 mcg (IV).
• In the case of upper airway obstruction:
- Nebulization of adrenaline (adrenaline without sulphite): 5 mg of a solution 1 mg/ml All 20 min to the need;
- The nebulization of adrenaline does not replace the treatment by adrenaline IM, but can add to it.
• In case of bronchospasm: The treatment is first the injection of adrenaline IM. You can add the standard treatment of asthma (β2-agonist, ipratropium bromide: see Mémo 3 Asthme).
• In cases of infringement of Cardiovascular:
- Raise the legs (if possible);
- The treatment is first administration of adrenaline im ;
- Filling vascular NaCl 0.9% 20 ml/kg on 10-20 min. To repeat to the need.
• In the case of shock refractory, consideration may be given to start an infusion in continuous of adrenaline. The starting dose is 0.1 mcg/kg/min, it should be titrated depending on the clinical response.
• Other treatments of the allergic reaction:
- Corticosteroids PO or IV/IO in function of the State clinic;

- Antihistamine PO.

Think About It

The Adrenaline IM is the basis of the basic salary of the anaphylaxis. Its rapid administration improves the prognosis and decreases the risk of a biphasic reaction.

Memo 25
Burns

I ♦ Definition
The burn is a tissue destruction brutal of origin thermal, chemical or electrical. In paediatrics, the burn the most frequent is due to hot liquids.

II ♦ Signs

♦ superficial burn
• Pain.
• Erythema without phlyctène.

♦ second-degree burn
• 2e superficial degree: erythema with blistering, pink background, red.
• 2e degree profound: erythema with blistering, brown background, whitish area, sharp pain.

♦ third degree burn
• The skin is cardstock, white or brownish.
• The location of the burn is insensitive.

♦ signs of severity of burns to 2e and 3e degree (do not count the 1st degree)
• > 10 % of total body surface (TBS)
≥ 5% TBS in infants < 1 year of age.
Or:
• Age < 3 years.
• Location: face, the external genitalia, soles of the feet, the palms of the hands.
• Any burn deep.
• Electrical burns or chemical, linked to an explosion or a fire.
• Circumferential burn.
• Suspicion of abuse.

III ♦ Supported in préhospitalier
• If intervention < 20 minutes after the burn, think to cool the skin.
• Calculate the surface of burns (in the Child, "the rule of the 9 "does not apply): see Mémo 1.

♦ Monitoring
• Prevent the cooling: remove wet clothing of the Child (+/- coverage of survival).
• Monitoring (cf, FR, SpO2, NBP).
• Measurement of the temperature → recheck if supported extended.
• Measurement of the blood glucose → recheck if supported extended.
• Evaluation of the Pain (Evendol from 0 to 7 years and then self-assessment for the older).
• Install VVP → if burns > 10% or significant pain.
• Sterile dressings of burned areas after rinsing in sterile water and application of dressings of hydrogel if available. Think to take photos (anonymity and family permission) before doing the dressings to avoid remove the dressings as soon the arrival to emergencies.
• Oxygen in the MHC → If the burn is associated with the inhalation of smoke of fire (measurement of HbCO if possible).
• If suspicion of burns of the airway (eyebrows, nose hairs burned, burns to face, hoarseness, stridor, soot in the mouth, difficulty breathing) → consider an early intubation (the majority of burns to face caused by hot liquids do not require intubation). In the case of the presence of soot, request the opinion of a Pediatric ENT in view of a fibroscopie with washing.
• If burns associated with an explosion → Do not forget to assess possible traumatic injuries (see Mémo 21 Polytraumatisé).
• If burning of the perineum or the genital organs → Ask a urinary probe early.

♦ analgesia
Favor a analgesia in the patient in now a spontaneous ventilation.
• Paracetamol IV: 15 mg/kg

• Morphine : dose of load: 50 to 100 mcg/kg then 25 mcg/kg in titration.
• Nitrous oxide (equimolar mixture oxygen-nitrous oxide). This mixture is anxiolytic and provides analgesia of surface after 3 minutes of inhalation; can be associated to the distraction.
In the absence of track IV:
• Ketamine : 5 to 10 mg/kg in IR.
• Nalbuphine : 400 mcg/kg in IR.

Fill ♦

• Any child Brulé > 10% of TBS should be infused.
• For the grand child: B21 (Ringer lactate) except if burns > 25%: filling at the physiological serum.
• For the infant:
- If normoglycémie : physiological serum;
- If hypoglycaemia: physiological serum + G10% in Y.

1. Calculation of the Body Surface Area (SC):

$$\frac{4 \times poids\ (kg) + 7}{poids\ (kg) + 90} = surface\ corporelle\ en\ m^2$$

2. Then calculate the basic needs for the child: 2 000 ml/m2 of SC/24 h.
And the added to the fluid needs to compensate for the burns: 5 000 ml/m2 of burned SC/24 h. Calculate the % surface burned to the 2e and 3e degrees (exclude the 1 degree). In the emergency, to assist in the calculation of the surface burned, there is a free application for Smartphones: "E-burn".
3. Divide the total by 24 to obtain a flow rate in ml/h, go half in the first 8 h.
For the short routes (< 1 h), we can consider simplifying the calculation in administering the solute of filling at a flow rate of 10 ml/kg/h for the first hour.

♦ suspicion of intoxication to cyanides
CYANOKIT® 70 mg/kg in IVL in 15 min (max. dose : 5 g).

Attention ! The administration of CYANOKIT® disrupts the blood balance sheets: think to make a levy before its administration if possible.

♦ Orientation
• If simple burns → transfer to an emergency service in order to allow a proper assessment by a specialist doctor. The evaluation in specialized center optimizes the supported.

• If serious burns → direct the child toward a resuscitation specialized for the Great Burned. Do not begin the antibiotic from the outset.

Memo 26
Septic shock/purpura fulminans

I ♦ Definition
The ˢᵉᵖᵗⁱᶜ ˢʰᵒᶜᵏ combines an infectious etiology and a state of shock. It is a serious condition which must be rapidly detected to prevent a mortality, morbidity.

The purpura fulminans is an extremely serious of invasive infection.

II ♦ Signs
Severe Sepsis marked by:
- Fever often > 39o ;
- An alteration of the general state: pallor, dyed gray, altered consciousness, irritability, abatement, lethargy;
- Headache, vomiting;
- Purpura: item necrotic or ecchymotique of diameter ≥ 3 mm. The purpuriques spots are not cleared to the vitropression and spread quickly in size and number;
- State of Shock: tachycardia, shallow breathing, elongation (> 3 s) of the TRC, cold extremities or cyanotic, hypotension;
- Among the child, the arterial hypotension is a late sign of shock, he should not wait for its appearance to recognize the gravity of the situation. On the contrary, the tachycardia is an early sign and evocative of the shock.

III ♦ Supported in préhospitalier
* Port of mask and gloves.
* Strip fully the child in search of purpuriques spots.
* Enclose the lesions to the pen in order to assess the character extensive.
* Monitoring (HR, NBP, FR, SpO2).
* Measurement of the blood glucose, lactate.
* Measurement of the temperature.
* Oxygen therapy.
* Fitting 2 VVP if possible.

* In case of failure, install an intra-bone.

IV ♦ Processing

* Antibiotic therapy started as soon as possible, even in the absence of levies:
- Cefotaxime : 50 mg/kg/6h.
Or
- Ceftriaxone : 50 to 100 mg/kg.
* Filling: 20 ml/kg of physiological serum on 20 min.
* After the second filling:
- Noradrenaline : 0.1 to 10 mcg/kg/min in grading of 0.2 In 0.2 mcg.
- +/- dobutamine 10 to 20 mcg/kg/min depending on the clinical criteria ultrasound or.

Think About It

Strip down fully the child (also remove the layer) to evaluate clinically.

Memo 27
Diarrhea and dehydration

I ♦ Definition
Diarrhea is defined by an increase in the number of the frequency of stools per day (> 3/i) and water content (> 80%).

II ♦ Signs
• Weight loss < 5 - 10% >.
• Moderate Dehydration:
- Reduced urine and dark;
- Eyes hollow;
- Dry mucous membranes.
• +/- fever.
• +/- vomiting associated.
• +/- abdominal pain associated.

♦ signs of seriousness
• Infants < 6 months.
• Severe dehydration:
- Intense thirst;
- Hypotension;
- Disturbances of consciousness ;
- Weight loss > 10%;
- TRC > 3 seconds.
• Associated malnutrition.
• Presence of blood in the stool.

III ♦ Supported in préhospitalier
• Weigh the child if possible (otherwise look for the last weight in the health record book).
• Examination:
- Ask the parents on the aspect of the stool: afécales, presence of blood in the stool;
- Duration and evolution of diarrhea;

- Concept of recent travel in tropical countries or contage (family, middle of custody).
* Strip down the child, make a full clinical examination (skin condition, mottled, skin fold, TRC).
* Monitoring (NBP, FC, FR, SpO2).
* Measure the temperature.
* Measure blood glucose.
* Install VVP if oral rehydration impossible. The oral rehydration can be done in some children with the help of a gastric tube and the administration regular or continuous basis solute from oral rehydration (SRO).
* Installation of IO if failure of VVP.
* Evaluation of the pain.
* Monitoring of the diuresis.

IV ♦ Processing
* Weight loss < 5%: solute from oral rehydration (dilution and conservation According to the SRO used). Frequent inputs and by small quantities (chilled if possible) of 30 to 40 ml in the bottle or in the syringe.
* Weight loss between 5 and 10%: oral rehydration or IV: B26 (4 g/L NaCl).
* Weight loss > 10%: rehydration IV.
* If hypovolemic shock: filling with physiological serum 20 ml/kg in 20 min. To repeat to the need.
* Antipyretics if fever.
* The anti-diarrheal are not recommended in the child.

Think About It

Think about the other causes of severe dehydration: kidney, adrenal glands, diabetes...

Memo 28
Electrified

I ♦ Definition

The electrifying is defined by the passage of an electric current through the body. It is necessary to distinguish the electric shock caused by a current at low voltage and that induced by a current at high voltage, the intensity of the voltage varies according to the electrical source.

II ♦ Signs

According to the Act of Joule, more contact with the source of current is long, more tissue damage will be important. The tetany caused by the current can lengthen the time of contact. The duration of contact increases the risk of ventricular fibrillation.

Intensity of the current (milliamps, mA)	Clinical signs
1-10	Tingling, twitch
10-20	Tetany
20	Threshold of release
20-50	Respiratory arrest
50-100	Ventricular Fibrillation
1000	Immediate ACR
> 1 000	Destruction nervous centers

I. Claudet, electrifying of the Child, Emergencies, 2009

• Electrical burns (among the child, the achievement of the hands and the achievement oral-lip are the most frequent).
• Disorders of the PACE and the cardiac conduction.
• Lesion of the organs located on the route of the current (until proof to the contrary, any child electrified has lesions deep).
• Tétanisation muscle.
• Signs of an infringement of the nervous system: bleeding, thrombosis, cerebral edema, Hemiparesis, convulsions.
• Electric shock can be associated to a trauma by projection or fall.

♦ signs of seriousness

• Arrhythmia.
• Loss of knowledge.
• Voltage ≥ 750 volts.
• Transthoracic journey.
• Burns of the 3e degree at the point of entry.
• History of cardiac pathology.

III ♦ Supported in préhospitalier

• To ensure the safety and security of relief, cut the current or ensure that the responsible for exploitation (rail service, EDF) were called if it is a current of high voltage.
• Pay attention to the risks of on-Accident (presence of water, etc.)
• Undertake the maneuvers of resuscitation if off cardio-respiratory (see Mémo 9 Arrêt cardio-respiratoire).
• Research of the points of entry and exit.
• Monitoring (cf, FR, SpO2, NBP).
• Do an ECG (continuous monitoring of the ECG in the case of signs of gravity).
• Measurement of the troponin if available.
• Sterile dressings of burned areas after rinsing in sterile water and application of dressings of hydrogel if available. Think to take photos (anonymity and family permission) before doing the dressings to avoid remove the dressings as soon the arrival to emergencies.
• Measurement of the temperature.
• Measurement of the blood glucose levels.

* Evaluation of the Pain (Evendol from 0 to 7 years and then self-assessment for the older).
* Monitoring of the diuresis.
* Install VVP if intense pain or signs of gravity.

IV ♦ Processing
* Paracetamol : 15 mg/kg in IV.
* Morphine : dose of load: 50 to 100 mcg/kg then 25 mcg/kg in titration.
* Nitrous oxide (equimolar mixture oxygen/nitrous oxide).

This mixture is anxiolytic and provides analgesia of surface after 3 minutes of inhalation; can be associated to the distraction.

In the absence of track IV:
* Ketamine : 5 to 10 mg/kg in IR;
* Nalbuphine : 400 mcg/kg in IR.

Fill ♦
Any child burned > 10% of skin surface should be perfused (see Mémo 25 Brûlure).
→ The antibiotic is not systematic.

♦ Orientation
The child victim of electric shock should be observed in hospital (SAU or resuscitation in function of the severity).
→ If simple burns: Transfer to an emergency service in order to allow a proper assessment by a specialist doctor. The evaluation in specialized center optimizes the supported.
→ If serious burns: Guide the child toward a resuscitation specialized for the Great Burned.

Think About It

* Do not return in a non-secure zone.

* Put a cervical collar if suspicion of spine.

* Do an ECG quickly.

* Monitoring +++.

Memo 29
Fever

I ♦ Definition
Fever is defined by an elevation of the central temperature above 38 oC. In the absence of intense physical activity, in a child normally covered, in an ambient temperature tempered; this is only from 38.5 oC it is possibly useful to undertake a treatment.

II ♦ Signs

♦ signs of seriousness
* Child < 3 months (< 1 months bacterial infection highly probable).
* History:
- Heart disease;
- Immunosuppressive treatment, a disorder of the immune defenses;
- Sickle cell anemia;
- Adrenal insufficiency.
* Fever associated with:
- Hemodynamic instability (cf, TA, TRC);
- Anomalies of the staining (pallor/cyanosis);
- Purpura;
- Disorders of the tonus and/or of the alertness;
- Anomalies of Cree or the reactivity;
- Excessive agitation/irritability;
- Signs of respiratory failure and/or compensated circulatory decompensated Or;
- Eating disorders.

III ♦ Supported in préhospitalier

♦ Examination
- Date of onset of fever.
- Taking of an antipyretic.
- Signs associated (behavior disorders, vomiting, diarrhea, headache...).
- History of the Child (febrile convulsions, chronic pathologies).

- Strip down the child.
- Measurement of the temperature.
- Measurement of the blood glucose levels.
- Monitoring (cf, FR, SpO2, NBP).
- Check the skin condition during a full clinical examination (in search of purpuriques spots or petechiae does not whitening to the vitropression).
- Check the voltage of the fontanelle in infants, or signs of meningeal irritation among the child.
- Ask a pocket to urine (ECBU) if clinically indicated.
- Reassure the child and its parents.

♦ In the presence of signs of seriousness
- Ask a track first device.
- Administer an antipyretic (taking into account the antipyretics given above: hour? Dose? Deadlines?).
- Consider a fill of 20 ml/kg of physiological saline.
- In the case of severe infection, begin the antibiotic therapy.

IV ♦ Processing

♦ An antipyretic
→ does prescribe that a single antipyretic medication, no study having demonstrated the interest of alternating or a systematic association.
→ prescribe the antipyretic medication to Effective Dose:
- Treatment of first intention: paracetamol PO: 60 mg/kg/I in 4 taken, or 15 mg/kg every 6 h, without exceeding 80 mg/kg/i.
→ Contraindication: hepatocellular failure.
- Nsaids (ibuprofen, ketoprofen and derivatives arylcarboxyliques):
- For the ibuprofen PO: 20 to 30 mg/kg/I in 3 taken, without exceeding 30 mg/kg/j ;
→ Contraindications: In the case of varicella, renal or hepatic impairment. To avoid when of hypovolemia (particularly in the case of diarrhea and vomiting) and streptococcal infections.
- Exceptionally, acetylsalicylic acid : 60 mg/kg/I in 4 taken (risk of Reye syndrome).

♦ **antibiotics (in case of suspicion of purpura)**
Cefotaxime : 50-100 mg/kg/dose in IV or IO.
→ If not track IV/IO accessible, a dose of ceftriaxone 50-100 mg/kg IM can be administered.
Other antibiotic therapies in function of the particular clinical context.

Memo 30
Intoxications

I ♦ Definition
^{Poisoning} is the second cause of accidents of the everyday life of the child. In the young child, they are often involuntary and are most of the time by the oral route.
In case of doubt on the conduct, refer your regional Poison Control Center.

II ♦ Signs

♦ search for Toxidromes
* Respiratory State
- Bradypnée/Apnea
Rapid Shallow Breathing -
* Hemodynamic Status
- Tachycardia/Bradycardia
- Hypotension/hypertension
- Vasodilatation
* Neurological condition
- Agitated
- Coma
- Seizures
- Miosis/mydriasis wards
* Status Uro/tract
- Vomiting
- Diarrhea
- Ileus
- Urinary retention

III ♦ Supported in préhospitalier
If patient unstable → take charge of priority to the vital functions.

If cab → *see Mémo 9 Arrêt cardio-respiratoire.*

♦ Examination

- *What product? What quantity? Total conditioning and remaining quantity?*
- *What time?*

♦ /Accidental intentional.
* Beginning of symptoms.
* Drugs available in the House. Make the drugs with the child when the transport to the hospital center.

♦ taken in overall load
* O2 if necessary.
* Monitoring (FR, FC, SpO2, NBP).
* Measurement of the blood glucose levels.
* Measurement of the temperature.

♦ ECG.
* Install VVP if necessary.

♦ Paracetamol (Acetaminophen)
The main risk secondary to a intoxication in Paracetamol is a hepatitis that can lead to the registry or to death. The initial symptoms are non-specific (vomiting, nausea, abdominal pain) and can appear several hours after the crisis. Hepatic impairment late clinical: drowsiness, hepatic encephalopathy.
* Toxic dose: 150 mg/kg in the Child; 10 g in adults.
* Treatment: To consider the administration of activated charcoal if ingestion < 1 h and if the state of consciousness allows.
* Antidote: N-acetyl-cysteine should be started less than 8 h post-ingestion, if it is not possible to obtain a metering before this period, administer the antidote. If a dosage is available (reliable if fact ≥ 4 h post-ingestion, refer to the nomogram of Rumack).

Doses	Children < 20 kg	Children 20 - 40 kg	Children > 40 kg
Loading dose	In 3 ml/kg of	In 100 ml of	In 200 ml of

150 mg/kg in 15 min	G5%	G5%	G5%
Then 50 mg/kg IV in 4 h	In 7 ml/kg of G5%	In 250 ml of G5%	In 500 ml of G5%
Then 100 mg/kg IV in 16 h	In 14 ml/kg of G5%	In 500 ml of G5%	In 1 000 ml of G5%

Slow down or stop the infusion rate if Anaphylactic Reaction slight or severe (see Mémo 24 Anaphylaxie).
Transport to a center of supported pediatric. Transfer in resuscitation in function of the clinical condition. If hepatic impairment severe, consider a transfer to a center with a specialty in hepatology.

♦ Benzodiazepine
Alteration of the state of consciousness, ataxia, dysarthria, respiratory depression.
• Treatment: To consider the administration of activated charcoal if ingestion < 1 h and if the state of consciousness allows.
• Antidote: flumazenil : 10 mcg/kg IV, max. 2 mg. Repeat as needed cumulative doses: max. 1 mg in the Child, 2 mg in the adolescent. A infusion in continues can be started to 10 mcg/kg/h if necessary.

Attention! Do not use flumazenil in case of intoxication mixed, because it may lower the convulsive threshold. Do not use in chronic users, risk of weaning and convulsions. The half-life of Flumazenil may be less than that of some benzodiazepines, there is therefore the risk of relapse.
Transport to a center of supported pediatric. Transfer in resuscitation in function of the clinical condition.

♦ Opiates

Respiratory distress, miosis, alteration of the state of consciousness, hypotension, vomiting and more rarely pulmonary edema.
• Treatment: To consider the administration of activated charcoal if ingestion < 1 h and if the state of consciousness allows.
• Antidote: naloxone : 10 mcg/kg, can be repeated 2-3 min up to clinical effects.

Attention! The half-life of naloxone is short (20-40 min), the risk of relapse is important. If repeated doses are necessary, start an infusion in continues 10 mcg/kg/h and titration according to the effects.
Poisoning by synthetic opioids may require high doses of naloxone, doses can be increased to 20-30 mcg/kg.

Attention! in chronic users, risk of weaning and convulsions.
Transfer in paediatric resuscitation.

♦ Cannabis
Involuntary ingestion (per os) of cannabis in the young child.
Alteration of the state of consciousness, confusion, nausea, tachycardia, respiratory depression, loss of inhibition, hallucinations.
Symptomatic treatment.
Transport to a center of supported pediatric. Transfer in resuscitation in function of the clinical condition.

♦ Alcohol
Involuntary ingestion in the young child, then volunteer among adolescents.
The symptoms of intoxication, alteration of the state of consciousness, respiratory depression, vomiting.
Risk of hypothermia and hypoglycemia, especially among the young child.
Symptomatic, no antidote.
For the adolescent, screening of a disorder of consumption and risk-taking (driving, other risk behaviors).

♦ **Other intoxications**
Tricyclic Antidepressant, beta blockers, inhibitor of calcium channels, derivatives of quinines, etc.

Think About It

• In the young child, the ingestion of a single tablet can sometimes cause death in particular with the following products: hypoglycemics, inhibitors of calcium channels, beta-blockers, opiates, tricyclic antidepressants, derivatives of quinine, etc.

• Always suspect a polyintoxication in case of voluntary intoxication.

• In case of accidental poisoning by illegal substances in the young child (including cannabis), the evaluation of the social context is necessary, and a reporting to the CRIP (cell Départementale of collection and assessment of the information concern) is recommended.

Memo 31
Malaise of infant

I ♦ Definition
It is a malaise occurring unexpectedly and brutal in an infant of less than 6 months. The causes are multiple, including the clinical manifestation of the stimulation of the reflexes laryngés pharyngeal and of airway, underlying infection, a convulsion, etc.

II ♦ Signs

- Hypotonia.
- Paleness.
- Cyanosis.
- Loss of actual knowledge or assumed.
- Apnea, +/- bradycardia.
- Vomiting, regurgitation.

♦ signs of seriousness
- State of shock, hypotension.
- Respiratory distress, cyanosis persistent.
- Disorders of the Conscience, abnormal movements.

III ♦ Supported in préhospitalier
- Examination of the parents:
- ATCD: prematurity, gastroesophageal reflux disease, drug therapy, recent trauma...;
-- A circumstance of the malaise: symptoms at the time of the malaise, last meal, convulsions, fever...
- Strip down the child.
- Monitoring (cf, FR, SpO2, NBP).
- Appreciate the time to recoloration dermal (on the thorax).
- Measurement of the temperature.
- Measurement of the blood glucose levels.
- Extent of lactate if possible.
- 02 at MHC if signs of seriousness.

* +/- VVP.

IV ♦ Processing
* Treatment to consider if specific etiology suspected.
* Hospitalization is necessary even in the case of full recovery after the malaise, for a monitoring by monitoring and the realization of complementary examinations.

Memo 32

Unexpected death of the infant (min)

I ♦ Definition
The ᴹᴵᴺ is the death of a child less than 2 years of age, without major history, occurring during his sleep and which remains unexplained despite the postmortem investigations. As well, it is only after thorough exploration, including an autopsy, that a "Unexpected death" can be declared "Sudden infant death syndrome".

II ♦ Signs
It is a multifactorial accident (association of risk factors).
* Individual Factors:
- Age between 1 and 4 months;
- More common among boys;
- Background: prematurity, delay of growth in-uterine, GERD...
* Family Factors:
- The unfavorable socio-economic conditions;
- History of min in the siblings (attention if the death of the twin per min).
* Environmental factors:
- Winter peak;
- Tobacco feto-maternal and/or liabilities;
- Hyperthermic environment;
- Ventral position during sleep;
- Co-sleeping;
- Soft mattress and/or dimensions not adapted to the bed, blanket, pillow, lint, Tower of bed.
* ACR of duration is difficult to determine, late finding of death (period of sleep).

• *Gasp.*
* Electrical activity without pulse.
* Clinical Examination, Search:

- Hypothermia;
- Coloring/rash;
- Lividités, rigidity;
- Signs of dehydration;
- Voltage of the fontanels;
- Releases/vomiting;
- Signs of malnutrition;
- Signs of maltreatment (hematoma, trauma, hygiene of the child).

III ♦ Supported in préhospitalier
* Strip down the child.
* Installing the scope to assess the heart rate.
* According to the context, start or not a cardio-pulmonary resuscitation (see Mémo 9 Arrêt cardio-respiratoire).
* Perform a full clinical examination.
* Take knowledge of the information of the health record book (vaccinations, history).
* Examine the place of death (sleeping, environment, animals...).
* Examination: duration of the ACR, resuscitation if started before the arrival of relief, circumstances of occurred: bedtime and discovery of the Child, the time of the last feeding, possibility of taking of toxic, treatment sedatives, Type of heating...
* Parents may, if they wish, to attend the resuscitation of their child. Some studies have demonstrated that this could help during the mourning, on condition that a first aider or a caregiver remains to their sides in order to explain to them the gestures.
* Be attentive to the psychological state of the entourage, do not leave them alone. If necessary, take contact with the treating physician for the psychological monitoring of relatives.
* Be empathic, humanize the child in appointing him by his first name, the present to parents after having removed the medical equipment, their propose to take in the arm, dressed, LANGÉ in coverage.

IV ♦ Processing

See *Mémo 9 Arrêt cardio-respiratoire.*

♦ **orientation in case of death**

Take contact with the center of reference of the min of sector. All cases of unexpected deaths of the infant should be explored. It is recommended that parents accompany the child during the transport to the center of reference.

According to the legislation, the transport of a body requires prior to obtain the written authorization of the administrative authorities, which may differ from several hours to the transfer, and generate judicial steps very heavy for the entourage. This is why, according to the local practices, it is recommended to make the death certificate to the arrival at the center of reference.

It is preferable not to have recourse to judicial authorities on the spot. The judicial investigation will be a brake to the transportation of the body to the center of reference and it will not be practiced to medical autopsy. In effect, the judicial autopsies (medico-legal) Looking for a child maltreatment, but medical research are not precise and does not allow to establish a diagnosis (e.g. : metabolic disease, malformation, sepsis, etc.).

It must consider the obstacle medico-legal in the case of signs suggestive of abuse. In this case, the doctor must take contact with the Prosecutor of the Republic.

In other cases, if there is no significant signs of abuse at the outset (attention to the hasty interpretations), the situation will be assessed on a case by case basis, as well on the place of death to the hospital, in the light of the results of the first investigations (Has/service of professional recommendations/February 2007).

Think About It

Fill the main sheet of standardised intervention at the national level, this fact sheet will follow the child and will be integrated in the medical file.

In the case of the unexpected death of a twin, it is advisable to hospitalize the baby survivor, in order to monitor and to practice of potential reviews.

Memo 33
Drowning

I ♦ Definition
The drowning is a asphyxia due to an immersion or a submersion in liquid medium.
It is the second leading cause of death in pediatrics.

II ♦ Signs
• 4 stages of increasing severity:
- **Aquastress** : Not of inhalation, Anxiety Child, exhausted;
- **Small Hypoxia** : slight inhalation, cough, shallow breathing, crépitants, anxiety, burnout, hypothermia;
- **Large Hypoxia** : inhalation important, cough, cyanosis, disturbances of consciousness, hypothermia;
- **Anoxia** : congestion tracheobronchial, coma, and even cardiopulmonary arrest.
• Take into account the duration of the immersion.

III ♦ Supported in préhospitalier
• Monitoring (cf, FR, SpO2, NBP).
• Stripping, drying (coverage of survival, heating pockets-soon…).
• Opening of the airway.
• Aspirations of secretion to the need.
• O2 MHC.
• Consider the tracheal intubation if respiratory distress or if disorders of the conscience.
• Install VVP.
• Measurement of the blood glucose levels.
• Measurement of the temperature.
• Extent of lactate if available.
• Installation of a cervical collar according the kinetics (fall).
• Installing a gastric probe.

IV ♦ Processing

♦ **If hemodynamic disorders**

Circulatory Filling: 20 ml/kg of physiological saline. After 30-40 ml/kg, inotropic consider (noradrenaline: begin to 0.1 mcg/kg/min).

♦ induction in rapid sequence

- **< 2 years:**
- Ketamine 3-4 mg/kg;
- Suxaméthonium : 2 mg/kg.

- **> 2 years:**
- Etomidate 0.2-0.4 mg/kg;
- Suxaméthonium : 1 mg/kg.

♦ sedation relay post-intubation
- Midazolam 100 mcg/kg/h;
- Sufentanyl 0.3 mcg/kg/h.

♦ Orientation
→ Transfer to a service of pediatric emergency if child stable, aquastress.
→ Transfer in paediatric resuscitation if drowning with signs of gravity.
→ Transfer in hyperbaric chamber if diving accident.

Think About It

In the case of ACR, continue the resuscitation if deep hypothermia because there is a chance of survival after warming, return to the normal temperature.

In the case of prolonged ACR, discuss the ECMO (extracorporeal membrane oxygenation).

Memo 34
Resuscitation of the new-born

I ♦ Definition
Approximately 10 per cent of new-born, any term confused, require a support to the transition ectopic.
For 1 per cent of them, of real measures of resuscitation are necessary to this adaptation.

II ♦ aid in the adaptation to the extrauterine life
• A alveolar ventilation effective started in ambient air in the new-born at term or with a FiO2 between 21 and 30% in the premature simply the more often. It is started, in all cases, before the end of the 1st minute, depending on the algorithm below. During the resuscitation, normothermia is maintained, the aseptic technique is respected, hypoxia and hyperoxia are avoided. If it has not been able to be anticipated, the request for reinforcement of the paediatric EMS is required.
• The ventilation is performed in positive pressure (VPP) using a BAVU or if possible insufflator with T-piece on first intent. If the pressures are monitored (Recommendations ILCOR 2015), they are commenced to 20-25 cm H2O, with a PEP to + 4 cm H2O, a frequency of 40 cycles/second. The first 3 breaths are slower: 2 to 3 seconds. The Chest must raise.
• The evaluation of the resuscitation is ensured by the heart rate and the figure of SpO2 to the right hand (position SUS-ductale).
• After 30 seconds of ventilation effective, if the CF is < 60/min, a effective circulation is ensured by chest compressions (CT) combined with the ventilation, with alternating 3/1, at the rate of 120/min. The chest compressions are performed in empaumant the thorax, the 2-inch joining to the lower 1/3 of the sternum, 1 cm below the line mamelonnaire. As soon as it has recourse to the CT, the FiO2 is increased to 100%.
• Endotracheal intubation is indicated in the case of the ineffectiveness of the ventilation to the mask, necessity of chest

compressions, of inefficiency or extension of the ventilation to the mask. It is also indicated for perform a tracheo-suction or if it is of a congenital diaphragmatic hernia. The gauges for SIT are in the table at the end of the sheet. The detection of the expired CO_2 confirms the position instillation of the probe.

• After 30 seconds, if the CF is always < 60/min, adrenaline (10 to 30 mcg/kg) is injected at best by a catheter umbilical venous non central (5 cm for a new-born at term with positive reflux).

• The adrenaline is prepared by making a dilution 1 ml = 1 mg of adrenaline, it adds 9 ml of NaCl 0.9% such that 1 ml of the solution = 100 mcg of adrenaline. It injects 0.1 to 0.3 ml/kg of this dilution. In the case of absence of catheter umbilical venous, the intratracheal instillation of adrenaline is still possible: 30 to 50 mcg/kg.

• *In the case of inefficiency of the resuscitation, the questions to ask are:* the technical gestures are they effective? Is it a hypovolemia (anemia)? A pneumothorax? Congenital malformations?

• In the case of acute anemia, is performed a fill of 10 ml/kg of physiological serum by catheter umbilical venous with urgent need of gall O Rhesus negative (15 ml/kg).

III ♦ algorithm for supported

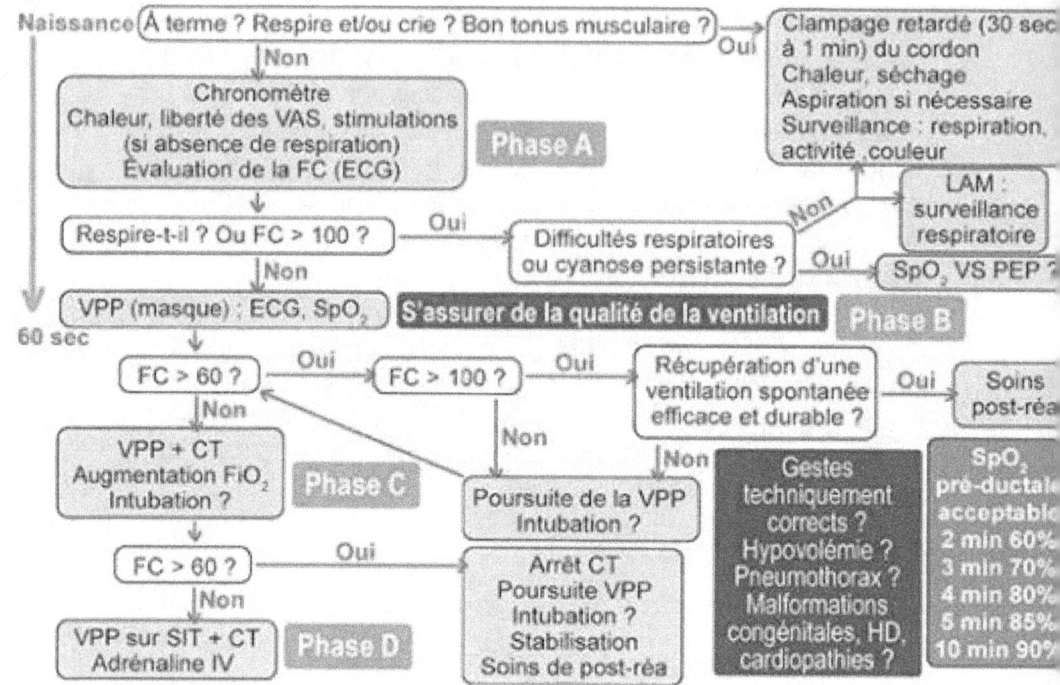

ECG : electrocardiogram
VAS : upper airway
Cf : cardiac frequency
LAM : amniotic fluid méconial
SpO2 : pulsed saturation in oxygen
VS PEP : Spontaneous ventilation in positive end expiratory pressure
VPP : ventilation in positive pressure
CT : Chest compressions
FiO2 : inspired fraction of oxygen
SIT : probe of the tracheal intubation
IV intravenous:
HD : diaphragmatic hernia

Particular case of the liquid méconial

• The presence of meconium in the amniotic fluid is the witness of a perinatal asphyxia. The new-born may therefore need to be resuscitated at birth if it does not breathe or if it breathes in an inefficient way.

In this case, the Phase A of the algorithm is done without delay during the 1st minute of life: suction of the oropharynx, drying, bonnet and stimulation.

• If a ventilation is necessary, it is started without delay after the aspiration and before the end of the 1st minute.

• Intubation is practiced only in case of obstruction tracheal in order to perform a tracheo-suction. There is not, currently, consensus on the way to achieve: intubation and suction through the probe of intubation, before reventiler or Tracheal aspiration with a large probe and then ventilation at the mask or direct aspiration on probe of intubation with withdrawal of the latter and réintubation for ventilation.

• If the new-born born in a liquid méconial did not need help to the transition ectopic, he will be just sucked in nasobuccal and monitored.

IV ♦ care and monitoring post-resuscitation

• Care and monitoring post-resuscitation adapted are performed: monitoring, CF, FR, SpO2, temperature, blood glucose levels.
• A gastric tube is asked to empty the air from the stomach. The Apgar score is reconstituted to assess the adaptation of the new-born and the effectiveness of the resuscitation.
• The child is transferred in neonatal resuscitation.

V ♦ Judgment of resuscitation

In the case of the new-born without Remaining Life (Fc = 0, respiratory movements = 0), the maneuvers of resuscitation are suspended after 10 minutes of effort of resuscitation continues and adapted.

There is no clear guidelines for all other situations, a notice is taken from the regional resuscitation.

Diameter of SIT according to the weight of birth

Estimated Weight of the new-born	Diameter of the probe	Blades of laryngoscopy
< 2 - 2.5 kg	2.5	Right Miller 00 or 0
2 - 3.5 kg	3	Right Miller 0 to 1
≥ 3.5 kg	3.5	Right Miller 1 or Oxford

Mark at the nostril = 7 + weight if nasal intubation
Mark at the upper lip = 6 + weight if oral intubation

Part 2
Equipment and techniques

>>> Mémo 35 - Attelle à traction de Donway
>>> Mémo 36 - Attelle cervico-thoracique (ACT) ou KED
>>> Mémo 37 - Attelles à dépression
>>> Mémo 38 - Bloc ilio-fascial (BIF)
>>> Mémo 39 - Capnographie/Capnométrie
>>> Mémo 40 - Ceinture pelvienne
>>> Mémo 41 - Collier cervical
>>> Mémo 42 - Cricothyroïdotomie d'urgence
>>> Mémo 43 - Damage control pré-hospitalier
>>> Mémo 44 - Drainage thoracique
>>> Mémo 45 - Électrocardiogramme (ECG)
>>> Mémo 46 - Incubateur de transport
>>> Mémo 47 - Immobilisation sur un plan dur
>>> Mémo 48 - Intubation
>>> Mémo 49 - Intubation difficile
>>> Mémo 50 - Matelas immobilisateur à dépression (MID)
>>> Mémo 51 - Oxygénothérapie
>>> Mémo 52 - Position latérale de sécurité (PLS)
>>> Mémo 53 - Procédures de radiotéléphonie
>>> Mémo 54 - Relevage à trois équipiers et à quatre équipiers

>>> Mémo 55 - Surveillance pendant le transport

>>> Mémo 56 - Ventilation au masque

>>> Mémo 57 - Ventilation mécanique

>>> Mémo 58 - Ventilation non invasive

>>> Mémo 59 - Voie intra-osseuse

>>> Mémo 60 - Voie ombilicale

>>> Mémo 61 - Voie veineuse en jugulaire externe

>>> Mémo 62 - Voie veineuse périphérique

Memo 35
Splint to traction of Donway

I ♦ Definition

The splint of paediatric Donway is indicated on the *fractures of the femur* (fracture of the femoral diaphysis).

It immobilises the femur and maintains traction.

It is contra-indicated if there is a trauma of the Ankle, foot, the basin or the lower part of the back.

If the two femora are achieved, the mattress of a capital property to depression will be preferably used.

II Technical ♦

Its implementation, at the request and under the supervision of the doctor, **requires three teammates.**

A crewmember maintains the basin.

A crewmember maintains the injured member in the axis by a progressive traction at the level of the Ankle, Foot Well stretched. It raises the injured member for the establishment of the splint.

The third crewmember adjusts the upper ring by dragging it under the knee and the dating back up to the top of the thigh, attaches the loop without the tighten. It prepares the splint in committing the two upper bars in the two branches of the "U" and in the Positioning to the side of the victim. It adjusts the length of the splint, puts to zero the dynamometer, loosens the clamping bars and raises the foot bracket, slides, the splint of hand and on the other of the Member traumatized. It urges the plugs on the lock ring in the upper bars, fixed the foot to the foot bracket at right angle by the bands self-aggripantes arranged in "8". It uses the pump to apply the pull pressure prescribed by the doctor, in general of 15 kg. The needle of the pressure gauge is located in the green area of the dial.

The maintenance of the member can then be released. The leg straps and leg must be adjusted, the clamping bars connecting the bars to the "U" must be locked.

It must finally ask the physician to check the correct installation of the splint.
The latter will not be removed to the surgical block.

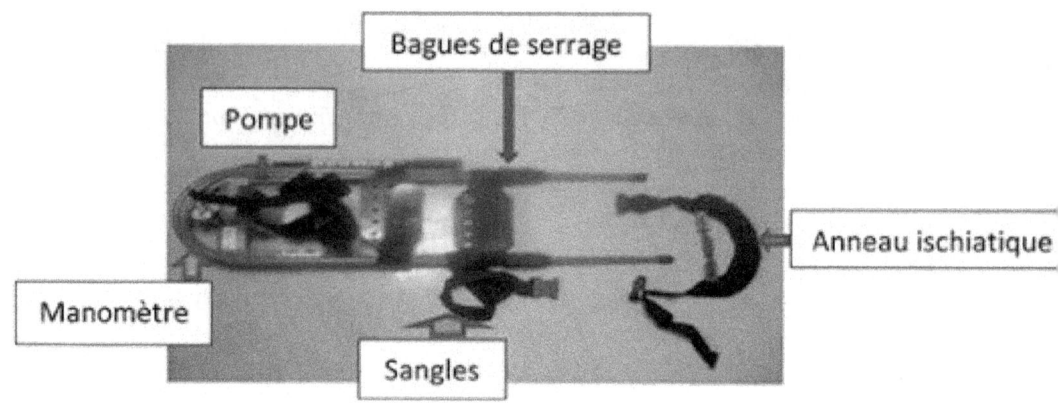

© L.D.

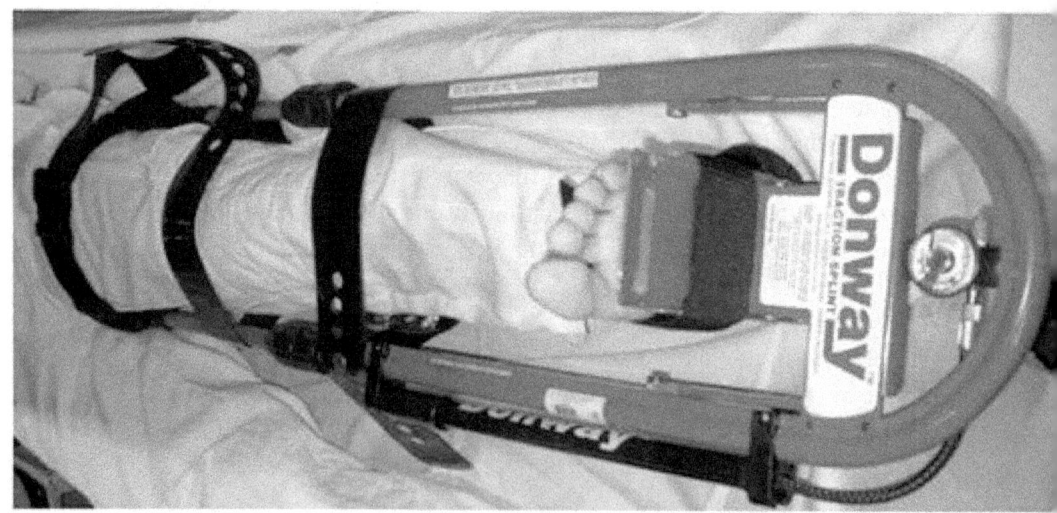

© L.D.

Memo 36

Splint cervico-thoracic (ACT) or KED

I ♦ Definition

Also known as *ked* for Kendrick Extrication Device, the splint cervico-thoracic is indicated to immobilise a victim reached a *trauma of the Spine* found in sitting position.

It Immobilizes the head, neck and back, and thus allows the installation of the victim on a hard plan or a mattress to depression.

II Technical ♦

After having put a cervical collar to the victim, as its implementation **requires three teammates.**

A crewmember placed behind the victim maintains its head during the entire maneuver.

The other two teammates are placed from hand and on the other of the victim: they take off slightly the victim of the seat and one of the two inserts the act between the back of the victim and the folder of the seat. They center The Act on the axis of the vertebral column, bring the victim to the contact of the Act, then slide the mobile parts of the corset under the arm of the victim and then maintain the thoracic corset by attaching the strap of the chest of the middle, upper and lower. They attach the straps of the thighs, passing under the latter.

They shake then the whole of the straps. They fill, if necessary, the space located between the band of head and the posterior part of the head of the victim with the cushion folded. They maintain the bands on each side of the head by two straps: one of the straps support takes on the forehead and the other under the chin on the high side and rigid cervical collar. The Maintenance head can be finally released.

Once locked, the victim must be lengthened on a hard plan or a mattress to depression. It will be entered by the handles of the Act and the lower limbs by two teammates.

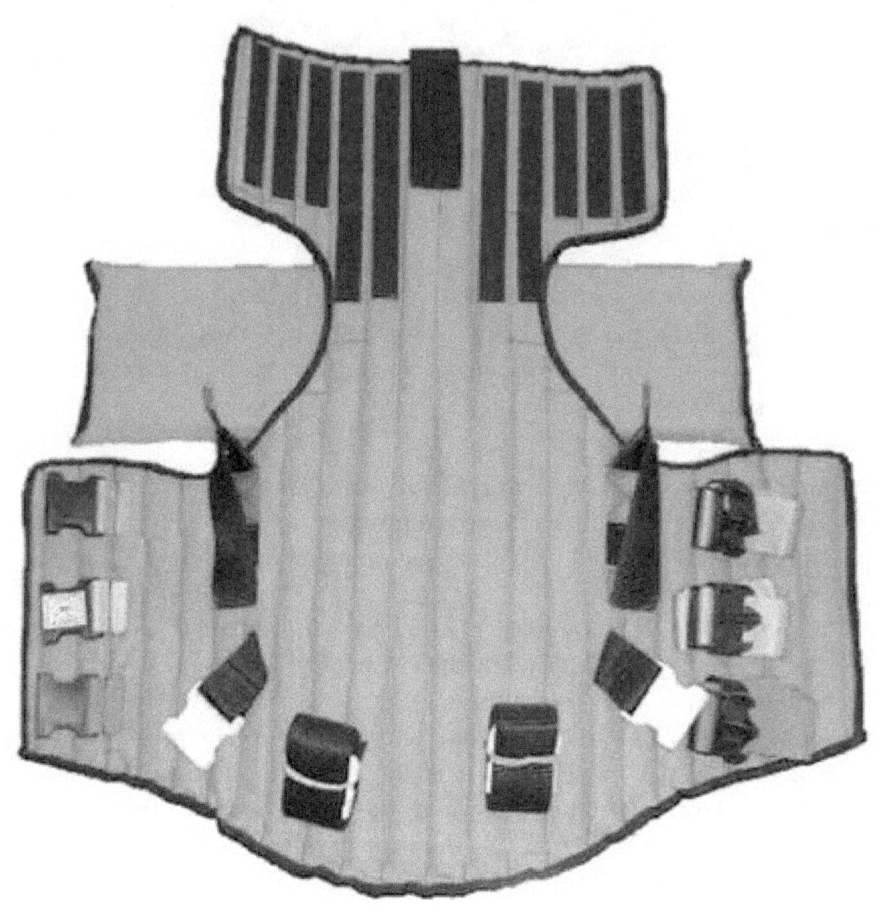

© L.D.

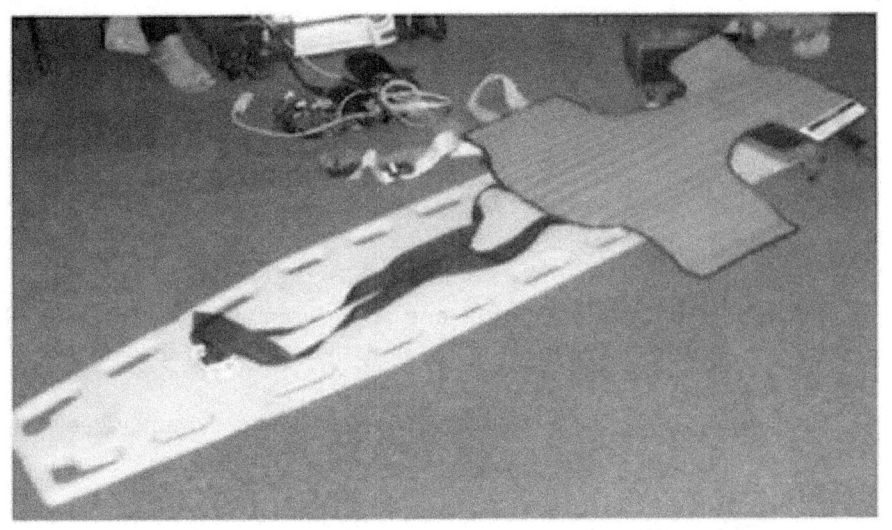

© L.D.

Memo 37

Vacuum splints

I ♦ Definition
The *splints to depression* are used to ensure the immobilization of the elbow of the front-arm and the wrist for the upper member, and of the knee, the leg and the ankle for the lower member.
The asset limits the movements of a Member traumatized, decreases pain and prevents the occurrence of complications.

II Technical ♦
The implementation is carried out by **three teammates.**
Two teammates maintain the injured member, at the level of the Joint SUS and underlying the trauma until the establishment of the splint.
The third crewmember prepares the splint by distributing all the balls and opening the valve of the admission of the air.
The two teammates raise a few centimeters the member to allow for the passage of the splint.
The third crewmember slides therefore the splint under the traumatized member taking care to encompass the articulation SUS and underlying it.
The two teammates deposit the member on the splint and maintain.
The third crewmember Rabat the splint of hand and on the other of the member while the two teammates move their hands to maintain the brace against the member.
And finally the third crewmember fact the vacuum to the inside of the splint sucking air until it becomes rigid. It then closes the valve and disconnects the suction device.

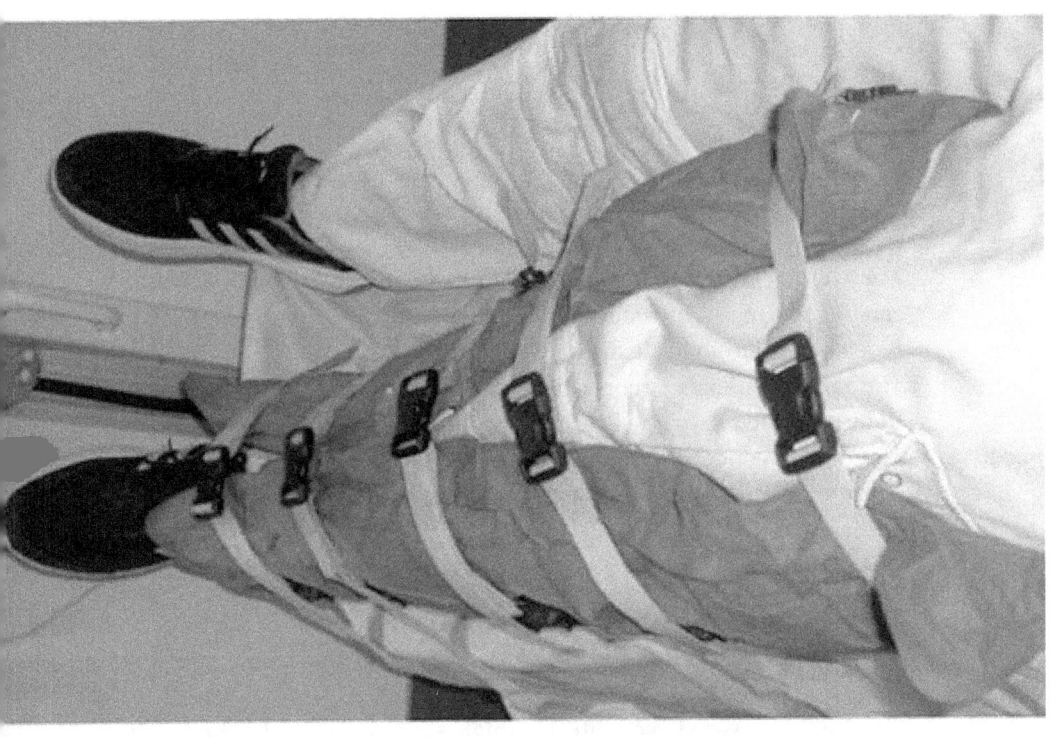

© L.D.

Memo 38
Bloc ilio-fascial (BIF)

I ♦ Definition
Anesthetic technique locorégionale device of the lower limbs that can be carried out by a doctor not anaesthetist.
Block of the Lumbar plexus by track earlier.
The Lumbar plexus is constituted by the previous branches of the Roots of L1 to L4.
The nerves concerned by the technique of the BIF are the femoral nerve, the cutaneous nerve on the side of the thigh and the obturator nerve.

♦ The femoral nerve
Mixed nerve sensory (and engine) to the anterior face of the thigh.
• **At the level engine:** flexing of the thigh on the trunk and the extension of the leg.
• **At the level sensitive:** anterior thigh + sides antero-the medial of the knee, the leg and the ankle.

♦ The cutaneous nerve on the side of the thigh
Sensory nerve.
Sensory innervation of the lateral part of the thigh.

♦ The obturator nerve
Mixed nerve.
• **At the level of engine:** adduction of the thigh (adductor muscles) + lateral rotation of the Hip (obturator muscle external) + bending the knee and medial rotation (muscle gracile).
• **At the level sensitive:** anesthesia of the internal face of the lower half of the thigh and the internal face of the knee.

II ♦ Indications
• Suspicion of fracture of the upper end of the femur.
• Suspicion of fracture of the femoral diaphysis.

III ♦ Contraindications

- Patient unstable.
- Deficit in G6PD.
- Porphyria.
- ATCD of PTH on the side traumatized.
- Cutaneous Signs premises (infection, wound...).
- Major DISORDERS OF HEMOSTASIS (AVK, haemophilia, severe hepatic impairment).
- Allergy to local anesthetics.

IV ♦ inguinal region
The inguinal region is comprised of:
- The Package vasculo-nervous: femoral nerve + femoral artery + femoral vein;
- Of the muscles couturiers outside and pectiné inside;
- At the top of the **inguinal ligament** extending from the pubic tubercle to the anterior superior iliac spine;
- At the bottom of the inguinal fold.

The region is covered by the **fascia iliaca** or aponeurosis of the psoasiliaque muscle, and then of the **fascia lata** or femoral fascia.

V ♦ technique of BIF

♦ **Hardware**

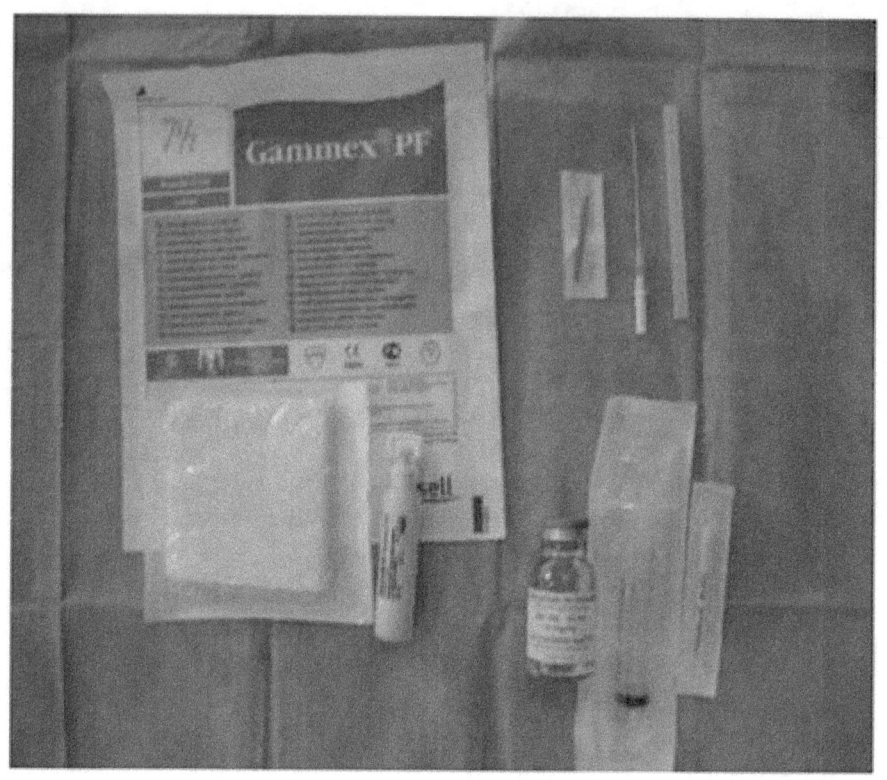

© L.D.
- Needle Short Bevel with mini-integrated blade.
- Xylocaine® non adrénalinée 1%.
- Syringe 20 ml.
- Pompous + 1 needle subcutaneously.
- Compresses.
- Betadine yellow.
- Sterile gloves.

♦ anatomical landmarks
2 through fingers below and outside of the Junction external third/two-thirds of the inside of the line between the anterior superior iliac spines and the pubic tuber (representation of the inguinal ligament).

- Patient in supine position.
- Disinfect and locate the femoral artery to be well at a distance.
- Collect in a syringe 20 ml of Xylocaine® 1% and adapt it to the needle under- the skin: inject 0.5 ml subcutaneously after suction.
- Achieve an orifice at the point for the puncture with the mini-blade, and then adapt the needle to short bevel in the place of the needle under the skin.
- Piquer perpendicular to the skin up to the perception of 2 (Jumps fascia lata and iliaca).
- Check the absence of reflux and inject 1 ml/year of age of 1% lidocaine up to a total dose maximum of 15 ml (note the time of injection).

♦ **Serious Complications**

They are for the most part related to the toxicity of local anesthetics.

Their **time of onset** extends the more often a few seconds up to 40 minutes.

Attention. If the accident occurs during the Injection: immediate stop of the injection.

- Clinical signs:
- Shooting pain;
- Vagal malaise;
- Disturbances of consciousness, or even convulsive crisis with precursors such as tinnitus, hyperacousie, dysaesthesias péribuccales, metallic taste, logorrhée;
- Rhythm Disorder (hypotension, ACR);
- Allergic reaction.

- Processing:
- Symptomatic of the complications: cardio-pulmonary resuscitation if cab, treatment of the allergic reaction if it occurs... ;
- Specific: **lipid emulsion in intravenous (Intralipid® 20%)** : bolus of 1.5 to 2 ml/kg possibly followed by an infusion of 8 to 10 ml/kg.

Memo 39
Capnography Extension/Capnométrie

I ♦ Definitions
• *Capnography Extension* : registration and graphical display, in the form of a curve, the variations in the concentration of CO_2 in the respiratory gas during the respiratory cycle.
• *Capnométrie* : continuous measurement of the concentration of carbon dioxide expired in the gas of the breathing circuit with digital display.

♦ The determinants of the EtCO2
• *Cellular activity* : the CO_2 is a waste of the organization, it is a cellular waste fruit of the production of cellular ATP. The more the cells work, the more they produce CO_2, in the normal conditions aerobic.
• *Cardiac output* : c is the carrier of CO_2 from the cell to the lungs where will be eliminated the CO_2 by pulmonary by the breakdown of the patient.
• *Ventilation* : at the alveolar level gaseous exchanges are between the oxygen which Between in the cell and broadcasts in pulmonary capillaries and CO_2 which broadcasts of pulmonary capillaries to the cell.

II ♦ EtCO2

A. Definition
The EtCO2 is the measurement of the maximum concentration of CO_2 in the end of the expiry by infrared absorption. The latter is intended to reflect the PaCO2, slightly lower value for healthy lungs (approximate less good that transcutaneous Pco2).
→ gradient between PaO2 and ETCO2 if ventilation disorders/infusion.

♦ Capnograph sidestream (sidestream and Microstream)

Sample of gas sucked the ventilatory circuit by a vacuum pump to be analyzed.

>>> Capnograph sidestream

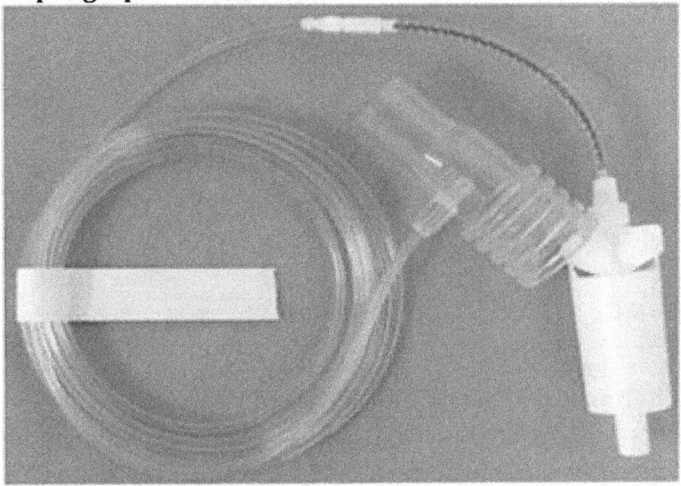

©A.M./N.L.

♦ **Capnograph non-sidestream (mainstream)**
Measure is doing directly in a small room, on the gas stream of the ventilatory circuit, allowing a direct reading. Can only be used in the patient intubated-ventilated.

>>> Capnograph non-sidestream

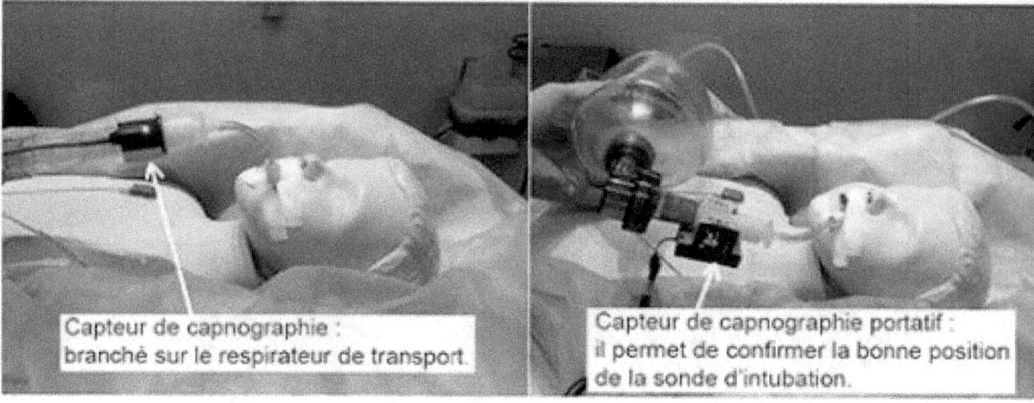

Capteur de capnographie : branché sur le respirateur de transport.

Capteur de capnographie portatif : il permet de confirmer la bonne position de la sonde d'intubation.

©A.M./N.L.

B. Interest and disadvantages

• Monitoring of the capnography extension:
- Allows you to confirm the correct position of the probe of intubation (may be in default in case of low flow circulatory);
- Allows you to assess the function of ventilatory continuously and non-invasive;
- Reflects the efficiency of the heart massage during a cardio-pulmonary resuscitation (low elimination of the expired CO_2);
- Allows you to detect the accidental extubation or disconnections of circuit;
- Enables the monitoring of the patient sédaté and ventilated and optimizes the supported respiratory.
• The use of a *Pediatric sensor* is necessary for a weight < 20 kg.
• The colorimetric sensors are unreliable in the child.

♦ **Disadvantages**
• Increases the space death.
• Monitoring the more distal.
• Sensitive to the presence of water vapor on the sensor.
• If respiratory rate > 30/min (FR normal for an infant): Capnography underestimates the value of the $EtCO_2$.

C. Technique

The sensor fits as close as possible to the probe of intubation, but after the bacterial filter (risk of contamination by the bronchial secretions), even if there is a minimal decrease of the reliability of the measure.

III ♦ TcPCO2

A. Definition
Transcutaneous Capnography: its measure allows to evaluate the function of ventilatory non-invasive manner to measure the rate of carbon dioxide in the patient (device coupled to the TcPO2 for new-born babies and to the SpO2 for children). It is the most used in neonatology.

B. Interest and disadvantages

♦ Benefits
- Reliability ++.
- TcPcO2 more close to the values of PaCO2.
- Delta less important than for the EtCO2.
- Does not depend on the ventilation/infusion.
- Not altered by the respiratory frequency.

♦ Disadvantages
- Period of monitoring more long.
- Risk of interference in the monitoring (Sensor incorrectly fixed).
- Risk of skin burn or eschar in case of prolonged Install (change the positioning of the sensor every 3 hours).

C. Technique
There are 2 types of electrodes.

♦ electrode TcPO2/TcPCO2
It is connected on a dry skin and clean:
- < 6 months: on the chest;
- > 6 months: on the anterior face of the forearm.
• Hyperthermia of the sensor allows you to increase the dissemination of gas, whose values depend inter alia on the temperature of the Electrode:
- < 28 Its = 41°;
- 28 to 32 Its = 41.5°;

- 33 to 36 Its = 42°;
- Term = 42,5-43°.

• It must wait approximately 5 minutes for a stabilization of the measure.

Attention!

The more the skin is fine, the more the temperature must be low:

namely that in these cases the period of monitoring is longer.

♦ **electrode TcPO2/SpO2**
It has several types of sensors:
- Mounting on the skin with sensor installed on the chest or the front;
- Or type clamp that attaches to the ear.

>>> Measurement Device PO2/tcpco2 type skin Radiometer®

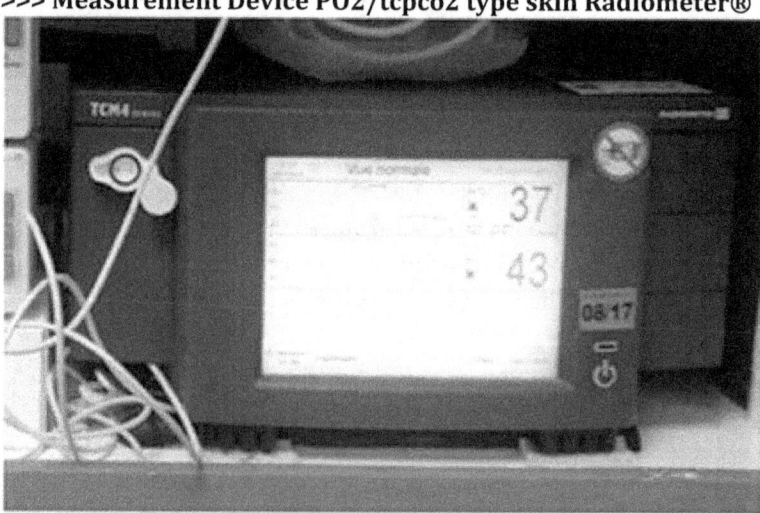

©A.M./N.L.

>>> electrodes with mounting on the skin

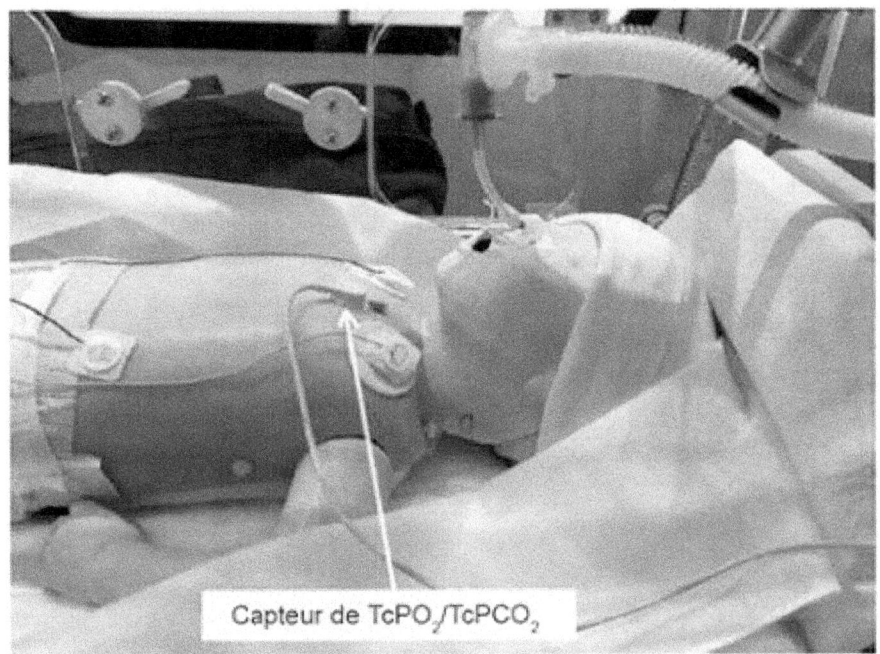

Capteur de TcPO$_2$/TcPCO$_2$

©A.M./N.L.

Think About It

The capno, this is not such as antibiotics : it must be "capno-tomatique..."!

• Mandatory when the realization of intubation.

• Continuous monitoring of the expired CO2.

• Mandatory when support for a cardiac arrest.

IV ♦ Standards
• EtCO2 = 35-45 mmHg.
• TcPCO2 : 40 mmHg (45-55 mmHg hypercapnia permissive"").
• SpO2 in the new-born between 92-95%. It must always be less than 95%, or even 92% in the premature < 32 Its because risk of toxicity of the O2 for the retina, the lungs and the brain.

V ♦ Monitoring CO2

The 4 phases of a curve of EtCO2 :
- *Phase A:* inspiratory line which is flat and 0.
- *Phase A B:* upward phase, it is the beginning of the phase that expiratory sign the emergence of CO2.
- *Phase B C:* phase of plateau. A phase of horizontal plateau is the reflection of a report Ventilation / homogeneous infusion.
- *Phase C D:* decrease in the concentration of CO2, the beginning of the inspiratory phase.

C = PETCO2

>>> **normal curve**

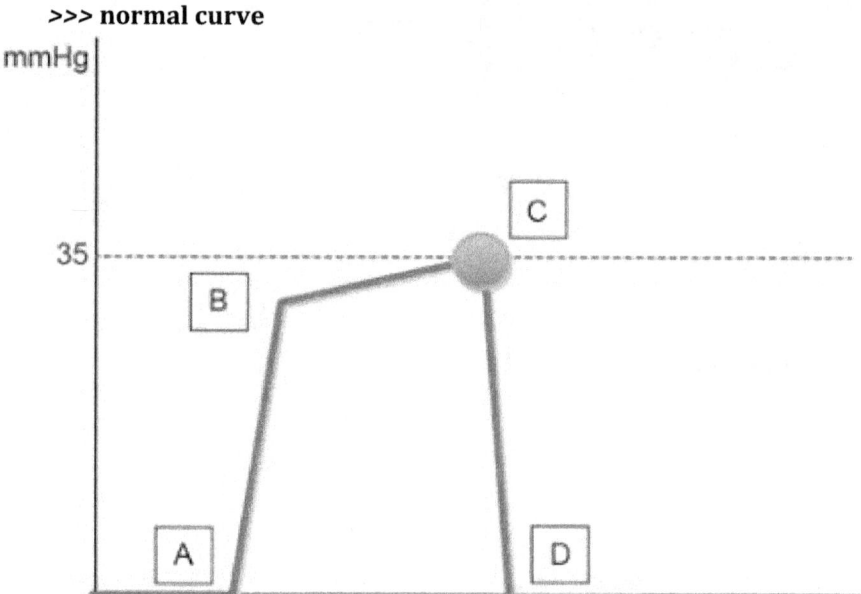

The *pelvic girdle* should be asked in systematic before any suspicion of a fracture of the basin.

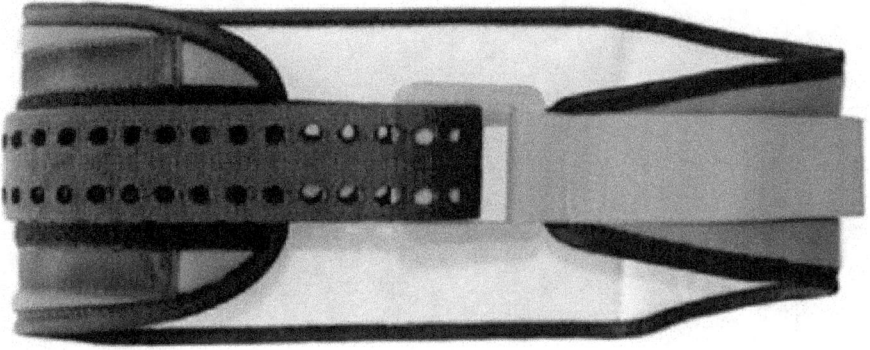

With the authorization of Medical Silvert

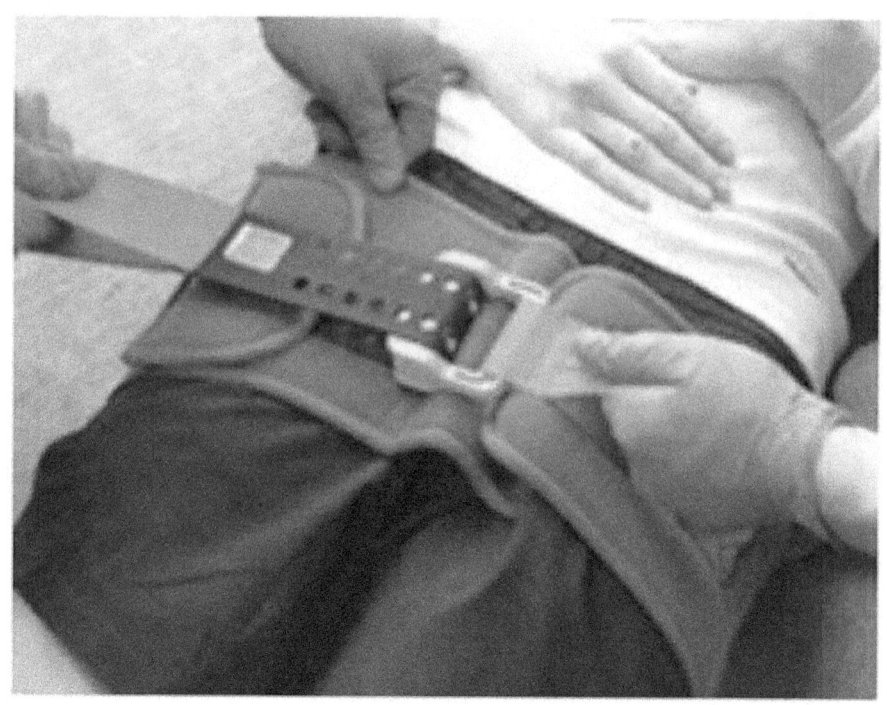

With the authorization of Medical Silvert

Of quick and simple to use, the belt **SAM Sling II** is equipped with a Loop" auto-stop" which hangs when the necessary traction around the basin is reached, according to the morphology of the patient (traction of 13, 15 and 18 kg).

3 sizes are available: X-Small, Standard and X-LARGE.

Its installation is simple and fast.

It will be withdrawn after notice radio.

Think About It

If you do not have this device, take a cloth and the position around the basin by performing a node for the Maintain or use the mattress to depression (MID) (but less effective).

Memo 41
Cervical collar

I ♦ Definition

The *cervical collar* is put in place as soon as a *lesion of the cervical spine* is suspected.

In response to numerous controversies, the cervical collar in the child is no longer systematically used outside of the extraction of the Child severely injured. The size must be adapted, as well as its positioning.

Source: advanced resuscitation neonatal and infant ERC 2015

The cervical collar is put in place after installation of the head of the victim in the neutral position and before any movement of the victim.

By restricting the movements of the cervical spine, it decreases the risk of onset or worsening of a lesion of the spinal cord.

II Technical ♦

Its installation requires **two teammates.**

A crewmember maintenance the head in a neutral position throughout the maneuver.

The second crewmember releases everything that may hinder the establishment of the clamp. He chooses a suitable clamp to the size of the victim or in Rule The size: the height of the cervical collar must be equal to the distance which separates the chin of the top of the sternum of the victim. It slides finally the rear part of the clip under the nape of the neck of the victim by releasing the or the bands self-aggripantes, and positions the front part of the clamp in order to obtain a good support chin-sternum before fixing the straps.

After the installation of the cervical collar, the head rest maintained up to the complete immobilization of the spine.

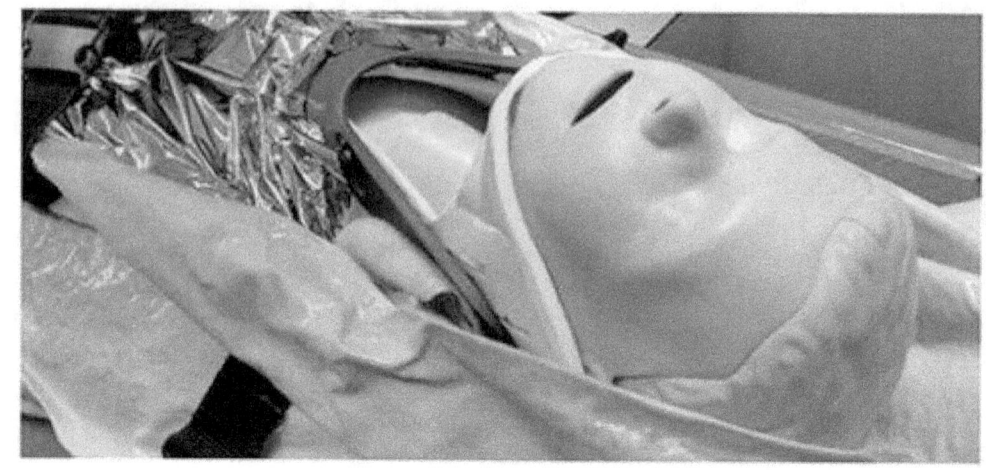

© L.D.

Memo 42

Cricothyroïdotomie of emergency

I ♦ Definition
The cricothyroïdotomie urgently to the Needle called "Fortune" allows you to ventilate using a catheter inserted in the membrane cricothyroïdienne. It is used in emergency when the other techniques of unblocking the airway are not effective. This technique is difficult to achieve in the infant and young child.

Risks: hemorrhage, laceration of the larynx, pneumomediastinum, emphysema, infection.

II Technical ♦

♦ Hardware
- Vacuum cleaner to the mucosities + probes.
- Resuscitation equipment nearby.
- Balloon to one-way valve (BAVU).
- Orange catheter (14g) newborn/infant.

→ beyond the infant:
- Child < 20 kg: There are kits of cricothyroïdotomie 2.0 bringing together the necessary equipment;
- Child > 20 kg: one kit adult may agree.
- Cobb No. 3 (adapter of probe of intubation) reserved to the newborn (malformations) or obstacle caused by a foreign body in the infant.
- 10 ml syringe.
- + compresses antiseptic.
- Plaster.

>>> **Equipment for a cricothyroïdotomie of emergency**

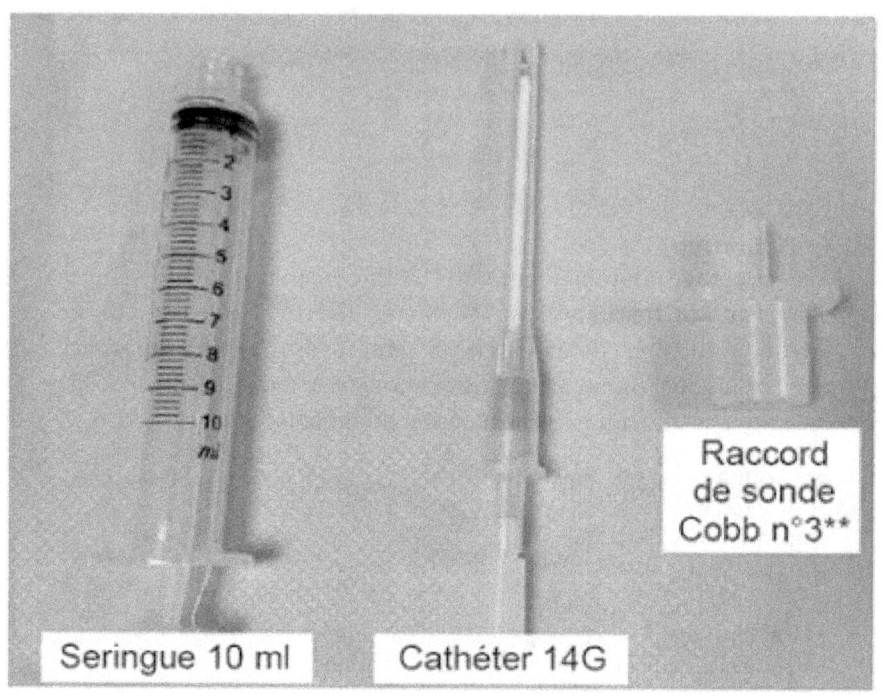

©A.M./N.L.

>>> kit of cricothyroïdotomie

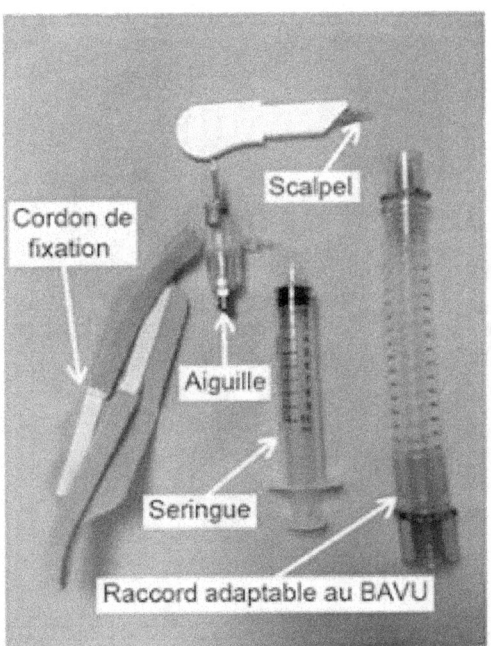

©A.M./N.L.

Technical ♦
- Good installation of the operator and of the child.
- Catheter connected to the syringe.
- Identify the anatomical landmarks.
- Disinfect the area.
- With one hand, stabilize the cartilage (cricoïde and thyroid).
- Stretch just below the cricoïde cartilage with a 45° angle in relation to the head (trachea under the skin).
- Aspire: the air suction confirms the good position, remove the mandrel.
- Connect to the Cobb of probe of intubation size 3 and a BAVU to ventilate manually.
- Attach the catheter.

>>> **technique of cricothyroïdotomie to needle**

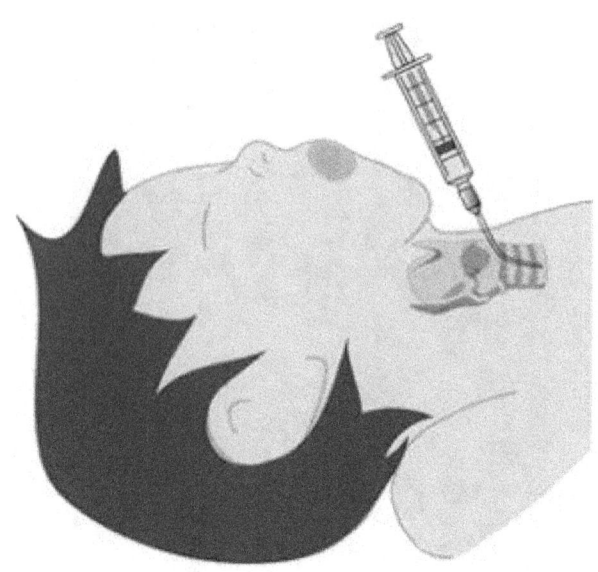

Think About It

With this method, the resistors are high, the volume low current, and the elimination of CO_2 is almost zero.

It is a temporary mode of ventilation to maintain a oxygenation, it must convert the cricothyroïdectomie or tracheostomy as quickly as possible by an ENT surgeon of pediatric preference.

Memo 43
pre-hospital care

I ♦ Definition
The Damage Control is derived from the military medicine. In the civilian community, it is used for children victims of trauma Penetrating or severe bleeding. It applies in a context of exception such as the attacks by firearms or explosives.
The aim is to maximize the chances of survival by carrying out rapid gestures, preventing the lethal triad (acidosis-hypothermia-coagulopathy) and ensuring a rapid evacuation to a hospital center for a supported surgery.

♦ Application of damage control **in a situation of exception with victims multiple Pediatric**
The major principles of the damage control apply in the context of exception, specially in the case of attack by firearms or explosive. In this type of situation, the rapid evacuation of patients is necessary both for the supported surgery, but also to minimize the risks of the teams on the ground (risk of on-attack). In comparison with the adult victims, children present more of Head Trauma or Penetrating wounds at the level of the head and may require more often a advanced support airway. However, the level of care offered must vary in function of the operational context and the degree of safety of teams. Only the essential actions must be posed, and a minimum of equipment should be used. It is recommended to constitute independent kits of damage control. It is sometimes impossible to monitor adequately the patient, some gestures will need to be carried out in the course of the evacuation, and gestures of advanced techniques (for example intubation) will not be able sometimes not be achieved due to the operational context.

II Technical ♦
The use of the doctrine *safe - Walking - Ryan* allows a prioritization of actions to be carried out.

♦ **Safe**

In a first time, arriving on the scene, use the mnemonic SAFE (borrowed from the military medicine) to ensure to intervene in any security.

Attention! Never intervene if it persists a risk for the team.

S	***Stop the burning process** - stop the threat*
	In the context of attack, the forces of the Order are in first line: sheltering or extraction of emergency medical teams.
Has	*Access the Scene* **- analyze the situation**
	Type of threat? Number of victims, gravity ? Communication between the different relief, authorities on Place: firefighters/UAS/forces of the order, etc.
F	***Free of danger for you** - Absence of dangers*
	Intervene and begin the care only in a secure area.
E	*Evaluate* **- Evaluation of the wounded**
	The first team on site is designated in the marshalling of the victims, the following teams support the victims and begin the walk: scale *jump start* for the sorting of the multiple pediatric victims ≤ 12 years.

>>> Jump Start

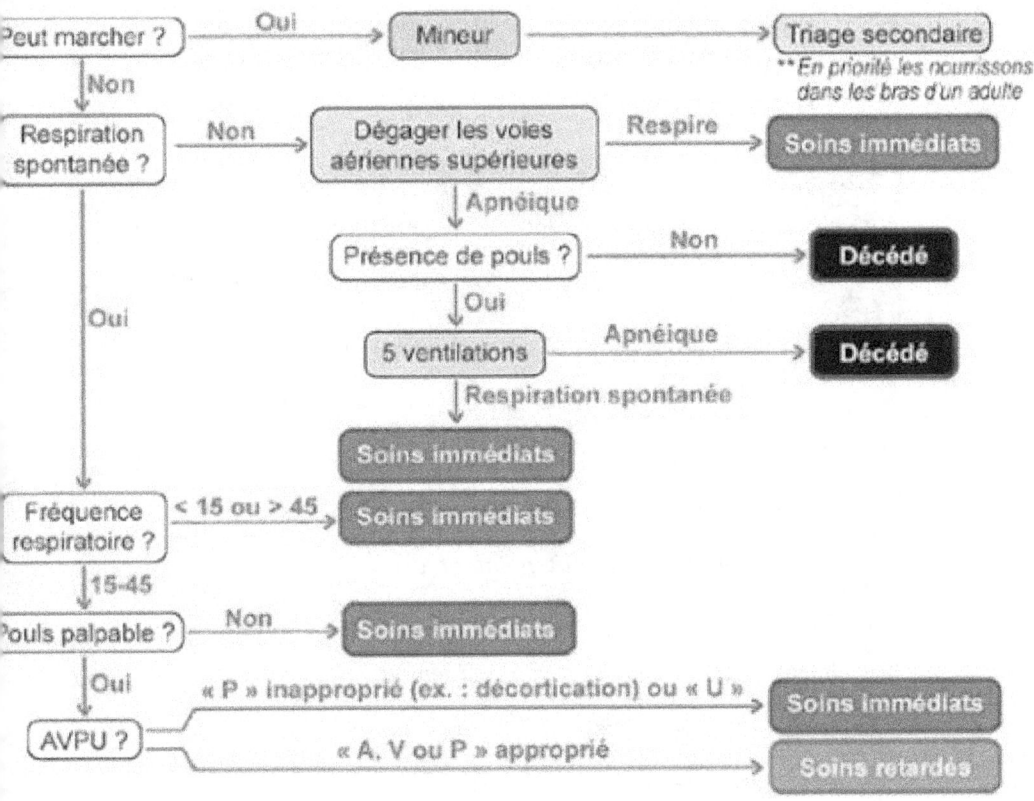

♦ **Walking**

The hardware present in préhospitalier must respond to the Algorithm *walk* specific to the support for child victims of *trauma Penetrating* or severe bleeding.

The teams must carry a *minimum of equipment* in order to allow them greater mobility in the framework of an operational context uncertain.

• Intervene with the appropriate equipment to the algorithm of damage control.

• Do not obtain the usual equipment of primary intervention: no monitoring, no vacuum cleaner phlegm, not of syringe, not a bottle of oxygen (the bottles will be issued by the PC logistics, depending on the context of intervention: explosive risk).

- The most simple is to equip of kits of intervention damage control in order to be able to "place" The walking quickly and effectively.

	Walking algorithm	Equipment
M	**Bleeding massive control - control of massive hemorrhage**	
	Strip the victim (this allows you to ensure that the victim is not trapped, Granada, explosives,...): Search of injuries in the *face and Dos, penetrating wounds with or without point of exit, amputations, bleeding, evisceration, burns, plague of the scalp, screening (children have more brain injury and penetrating trauma at the level of the head that the adults).*	• Pair of Universal Scissors Designed to cut all types of fabrics type Jesco®.
	Withers tactical (turnstile) or pneumatic tourniquet: it must be asked early. → In the young child, the pneumatic tourniquet of pediatric size is the withers of choice. The diameter of the tourniquets tactics may be too large for children < 8 years, however goldeneyes	• Tactical Goldeneye pediatric size. • Tourniquets tires (3 pediatric sizes). • Have a pen-marker on itself.

tactics of 4 cm in diameter are now marketed.

Technique of installing the tactical tourniquet

• Safety Screws dessérée (present on some tourniquets tactics), Handle of torsion in travel limiter.

• Engage the withers by the end of the member.

• The position at 5-7 cm above the wound, wide part toward the outside of the member reaches.

• Tighten the strap firmly.

• Screw the safety screws to its maximum.

• Turn the twist grip until the stop of the hemorrhage.

• Lock the handle using the triangle of maintaining the most appropriate.

• Note the time to install on the withers or on the front of the victim.

→ its effectiveness is determined by the judgment of the bleeding and the absence of pulse.

→ The withers must always remain visible: Monitor the resumption of bleeding (in which case a second withers will be installed upstream of the first withers without removing the first).

→ The objective is to remove the withers to the operating block in a period of 2 hours maximum.

Technique of installing the pneumatic tourniquet

The withers tire is composed of a pressure gauge, a pear and a cuff.

• Position the cuff and well tighten the tourniquet around the member upstream of the bleeding.

• Introduce the tube fitting at the stop in the quick coupler.

• Connect the cuff to the pressure gauge.

• Inflate the cuff to the aid of the Pear Up to reach the maximum pressure.

• Secure the whole by tightening the straps or twine (depending on the model).

• Note the time to install on the withers or on the front of the victim.

→ its effectiveness is determined by the judgment of the bleeding and the absence of pulse.

→ The withers must always remain visible: Monitor the resumption of bleeding.

If not from withers specific to provision, possibility to make a tourniquet of Fortune:

• Use a fabric, nor too late, or too thick (not twine, or cord), and a long object, solid and rigid, as a pen.

• Slide the first link under the member, 5-7 cm above the wound.

• Place the second link on the first and the long of the member.

• Tighten the first link.

• Place the wand on the node.

• Make a second node taking the protective strip.

• Turn the rod up to the judgment of

the bleeding. • The secure with the second link. • Note the time to install on the withers or on the front of the victim.	
Haemostatic Band: it allows you to fill a hemorrhagic wound prior to the establishment of a pressure dressing. The aim is to bring the band to the contact of the vein or artery which bleeds. It can be used in priority for the non-bleeding garrotables, penetrating wounds at the level of the chest, back, etc. • Insert the haemostatic band in the wound in the pull-down. • In function of the depth of the wound, possibility to use several hemostatic bands. • Cover the hemostatic dressing with a pressure dressing. • Note that a haemostatic bandage has been put in place in order to inform the medical teams following.	• Hemostatic Bands
Pressure dressing: it includes several	• Compression

elements on a same band loose, non-adherent *band. Its handle allows to use this dressing on the parts of the body not garrotables (head, neck, hip, etc.). It allows them to lead and to effectively maintain the band. Its position allows you to exert a direct pressure on the wound.	*compresses Bandages Dressings *Handle System
Plague of the scalp: use staples or wire to skin to allow in a first time to reconcile the edges and decrease the bleeding.	• Aggrafes and/or wires to skin
American dressings + bands: for the wounds, burns and éviscérations (circle the abdomen without tightening the band).	• American Dressings + BANDS

Has Airways - the airway

• Position the victim in order to release the airway. • Unclog the airway manually if needed. • If the victim is unconscious, put a	• Guedel (various sizes). • Cricothyroïdotomie: - Catheter 14G;

guedel. • In the case of airway obstruction linked to a facial trauma: Practice a cricothyroïdotomie of emergencies (see Mémo 42).	- Syringe 10 ml; - Cobb no. 3. • And/Or kit of cricothyroïdotomie 2.0 for children < 20 kg: Beyond, a kit adult can be used.
Breathing	
• Put the victim seated or half-seat in the event of respiratory difficulties.	
• *If O2 to provision:* put a mask to high concentration (minimum flow rate of 6 l/min: see Mémo 56).	• Mask to high concentration (sizes: pediatric, adult).
• If unconscious victim, needing assistance: ventilatory ventilate the Bavu (ball to one-way valve).	• BAVU pediatric and adult BAVU.
• *In the case of penetrating wound of the chest (blower wound):* Make a bandage 3 sides or use a valve of Asherman.	• Dressing 3 sides: Use a Packaging Type: laminated face of the package of compresses or two dressings of type TEGADERM® pasted

	the one on the other, and the plaster leaving one side of the Dressing open. • Or valve of Asherman.
• *In the case of compressive pneumothorax:* make a exsuflation to the Needle and if necessary in a second time ask a chest tube (see Mémo 44 Drainage thoracique).	• Catheter. • Syringe 10 ml.

C | **Movement** | |
|---|---|
| • Ask a track peripheral venous (VVP).
• *If failure:* install of an intra-bone.
(See Mémos 59 and 62). | • Equipment for installing a VVP.
• Equipment for installing a IO.
= Several sizes of needles. |
| • The indication of the blood pressure is made if perception of the Radial pulse or humeral (because not monitor to provision).
• *If Absence of pulse*: Start a filling: 10 | • Pockets of solutes of physiological saline. |

ml/kg on 20 minutes.

→ *In a second time, when the voltage can be monitored,* <u>blood pressure goals will be the following:</u>

	≤ 2 years	2 to 10 years
Neurotrauma	PAM ≥ 55 mmHg	PAM ≥ 65 mmHg
Absence of neurotrauma	PAM ≥ 45 mmHg	PAM ≥ 55 mmHg

Proposed by G. Orliaguet-Necker,

Adapted from Haque MCCPS 2007

- As soon as the second filling, consider a inotropic support: noradrenaline begin to 0.1 mcg/min/kg in PSE in the UMH.
- In case of bleeding or victims

- Noradrenaline bulb.
- Pocket of physiological serum.
- Ampoules of

considered at high risk hemorrhagic, begin rapidly Tranexamic acid (in the first 3 hours of Supported): < 10 years: 10 to 15 mg/kg on 10 min (maximum 1 g). > 10 years: 1 g on 10 min. **Caution:** risk of hypotension if injection too fast.	tranexamic acid. • Pockets of physiological saline. • Dilution 1 mg in 100 ml physiological saline.

H Head/hypothermia - **neuro/Hypothermia**

Hypothermia is a component of the Triad lethal. Among the child victim of trauma, it is associated with the increase in the Mortality (loss of 1°C = decrease of 10% of the functions of the hemostasis). • Cover the victim. • Remove wet clothing. • Isolate the ground.	• Blankets of survival.
Assessment of the neurological status of the victim. • Assess the symmetry of the wards. • Make the AVPU (see sheet polytraumatisé).	• Lamp.

171

E	Evacuation	
	• Among the child there is no specific means of evacuation: Protect in the coverage of survival, evacuate in the arm of a rescuer, otherwise evacuation on flexible stretcher as for the adult.	
	• Identify the victims with medical sheets of the front and bracelets sinus (allows you to trace the victim by giving him a identity thanks to a bar code and a unique number). • In order to allow the monitoring and to make the link between the members of a same family (example mother/child), paste the bar code of the medical record of the front of the A on the back of the plug at the other and vice versa. • Detachable part at the bottom of the plug to keep, the rest follows the victim.	• Medical sheet of the front and bracelets sinus.

Attention!

We must never go to the next item as long as the previous item is not controlled.

♦ **Ryan**
At the end of the first walking, if the evacuation Tarde, continue the procedure with the Ryan.

R	**Reassess**	
	Reassess each item from the walk: effectiveness of tourniquets, filling, permeability of VVP, mounting, etc.	
Y	**Eyes**	
	Monitor the neurological condition of the victim.	
Has	**Analgesia**	
	Morphine or ketamine (started in a second time).	
N	**Antibiotic therapy**	
	AUGMENTIN® (started in a second time).	

>>> **Types of tourniquets tactics (left) and tires (right)**

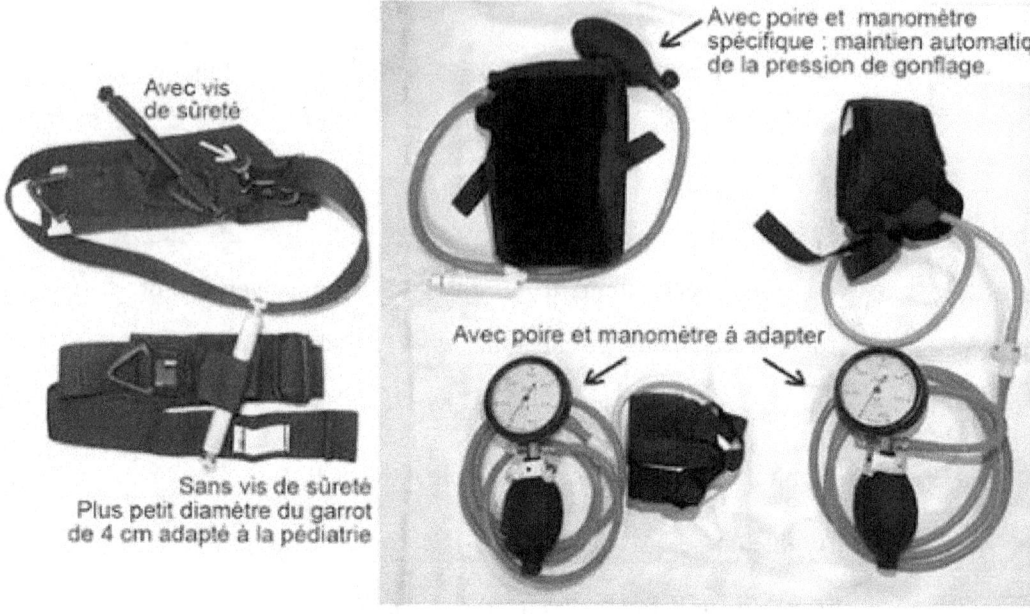

©A.M./N.L.

>>> Withers tactics with safety screws (left) and small diameter without safety screws (Right)

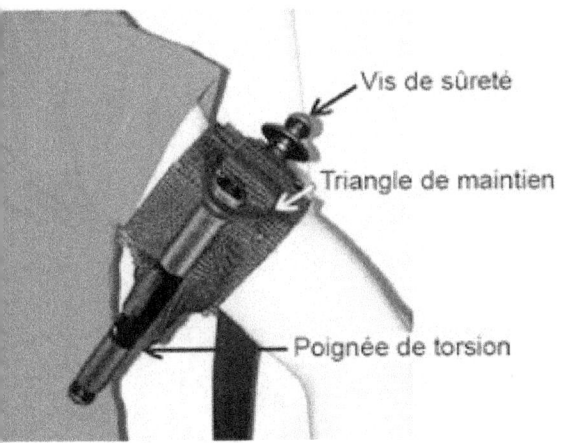
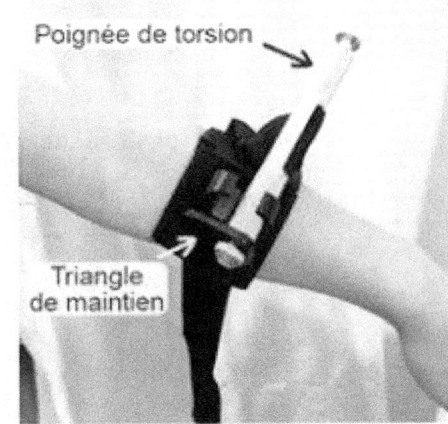

©A.M./N.L.

>>> **tourniquets tires**

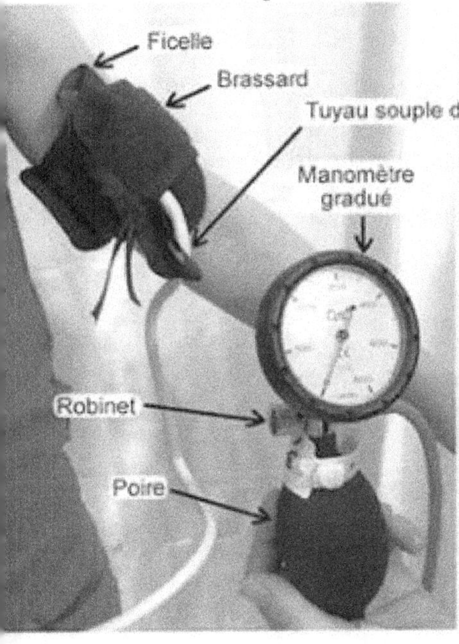

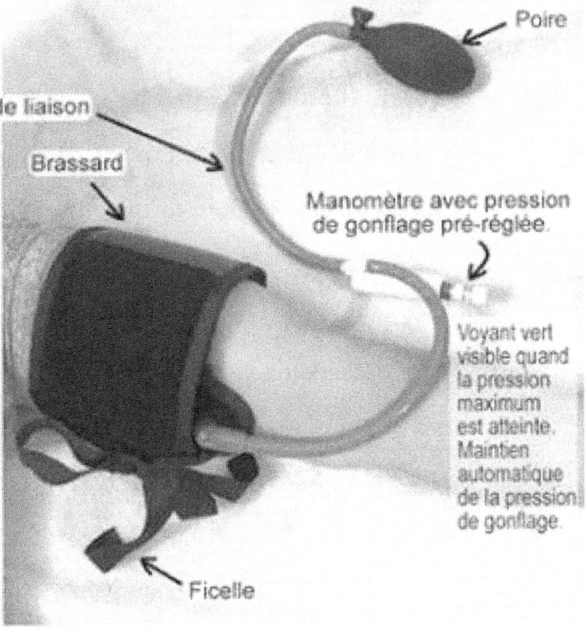

>>> valve for the Asherman

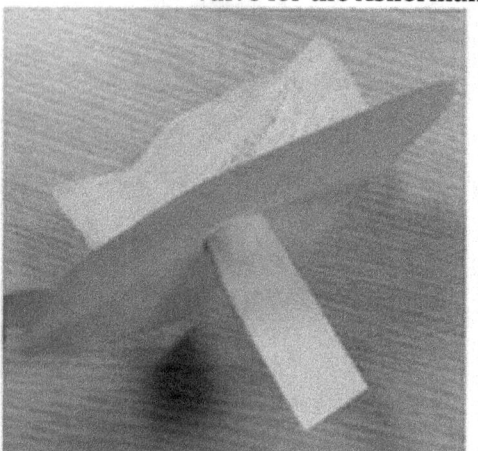
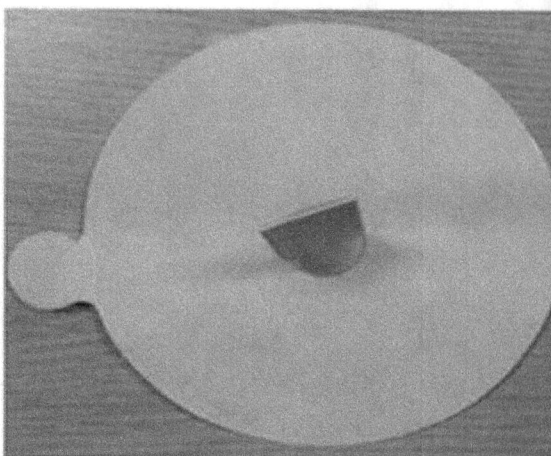

Think About It

• The kit should contain the material basis for the establishment of venous track and the disinfection of wounds: antiseptics, plaster, compresses, tubing, etc.

• Remember to wear gloves during the interventions particularly in case of bleeding.

• Do not intervene if the area is not secure.

• Possibility to equip the UMH (mobile units Hospitallers) of atropine and INEUROPE® in case of CBRN disasters.

Memo 44
Thoracic drainage

I ♦ Definition

In préhospitalier, the laying of thoracic drain is done mainly in case of suspicion of pneumo-/hemothorax. In the event of tension pneumothorax, the exsufflation To The needle should be carried out rapidly. A chest tube may be asked in a second time in function of the clinical status of the patient and of the judgment of the clinician.

Note: In neonatology, thanks to new ventilatory practices, the incidence of pneumothorax compression bandages to drastically decreased since several years. The installation of drain is become exceptional: the exsufflation is sometimes still necessary in case of bad tolerance and transillumination after (or even ultrasound or radiography in maternity).

II Technical ♦

A. Exsufflation to needle

♦ Hardware
• Box to needles.

• Compresses.

• Antiseptic.

• *The* needle or catheter connected to a cock 3 tracks (épicrânienne No. 22G or catheter for 24G in neonatology).
• Local Anesthetic of type Xylocaine® 1%.
• 10 ml syringe.
• Dressing of type TEGADERM®.

♦ **technique for the exsufflation to needle (simple pneumothorax or under voltage)**
• Resuscitation equipment at hand and source of oxygen. The patient must be under Monitoring Monitoring: ECG, SpO2, PA.
• Reassure the child.
• Identify the second intercostal space on the midclavicular line.
• Washing of hands, port of mask, Charlotte, port of gloves and gown sterile.
• Disinfect the puncture site on, anesthetize locally according to the degree of urgency.
• Connect the catheter to the syringe to prick in suction.
• Piquer perpendicular to the skin, advance the catheter to the upper edge of the 3e coast until the pleural space.
• The aspiration of air or the perception of a small noise indicating the outcome of Air Shows the good position of the catheter. S immobilise and vacuum the air.
• Once the suction made in the syringe, remove the catheter or the épicrânienne and make an occlusive dressing.
• Assess the clinical condition of the patient and the clinical response of the procedure.
• Assess if the patient requires the insertion of a chest tube following the procedure of exsufflation.
→ To Consider including if the patient remains clinically unstable, shows signs of re-accumulation of the pneumothorax, air transport is envisaged, etc. The presence of a pneumo/traumatic hemothorax usually requires the installation of a drain of the chest.

B. Install thoracic drain

♦ **Hardware**
• Box to needles.

• Compresses.

• Antiseptic.

• Local Anesthetic of type Xylocaine® 1%.
• Thoracic drain.
• Dressing of fixing of type TEGADERM®.

- Wire to skin.

- Scalpel.

- Unidirectional valve (valve type of HEIMLICH): Always use a single valve anti-reflux, do not associate it with a system of collection in suction of type PLEUREVAC®.

Or

- Suction system of type PLEUREVAC®.
→ during transfer inter-hospitalier the drain of the chest can be connected to a compendium of aspiration of PLEUREVAC type® which will regulate the aspiration to - 20 cmH2O: think of clamp the system during the mobilization of the Child and the déclamper when it is installed.

♦ **technique for the installation of the chest**
- Sunset the Child on the back, position his hand under her head to release the axillary region. The reassure. The patient must be under Monitoring Monitoring: ECG, SpO2, PA.
- According to the clinical condition, a local analgesia or analgesia by the intravenous route can be envisaged.
- Select the size of chest appropriate depending on the age of the Child:
- NN: 8-12 F;
- 1 Year: 16-20 F;
- 4 years: 20-28 F;
- 10 years: 28-32 F;
- > 14 years: 28-32 F.
→ For drainage of a simple pneumothorax, the smaller size of thoracic drain in function of the age may be selected. In the case of hemothorax or bestowal the upper size must be chosen.
- Identify the anatomical landmarks: 4e or 5e intercostal space at the level of the anterior axillary line (height of the nipple in the child Pre-pubescent).
- Washing of hands, port of mask, Charlotte, port of gloves and gown sterile.
- Disinfect the puncture site on, anesthetize locally according to the degree of urgency.

- Make a small incision of the skin using the scalpel.
- Advance the drain with the trocar in place (upper edge of the lower coast of the space) to penetrate the pleural space (loss of resistance, arrival of air or liquid). STOP and remove the trocar. Lead:
- At the top and in front for a air effusion;
- At the bottom and rear for a fluid effusion;
- At the top and rear if joint effusion (trauma).

Be careful not too advance in the pleural space with the trocar in place because the risk of pulmonary puncture or cardiac important. To help, use his fingers as a stop when the insertion of the drain.
- Once the trocar removed, move the drain in the pleural space up to the desired location.
- Clamp the drain until it is connected to a unidirectional valve.
→ Do not forget to remove the clamp as quickly as possible by the suite.
- Connect to a unidirectional valve and a system of collection for single use.
- Attach the drain to the skin using a wire and then a dressing transparent.

Be careful not to bend or crush the drain which would prevent the drainage in continuous.
- Regularly check the drain and the operation of the valve.
- When possible, a chest x-ray should be made to confirm the position of the drain of the chest.

>>> Type of drain the chest

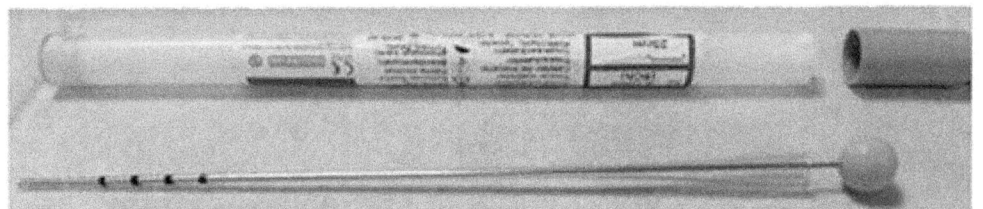

©A.M./N.L.

>>> Valve For Heimlich

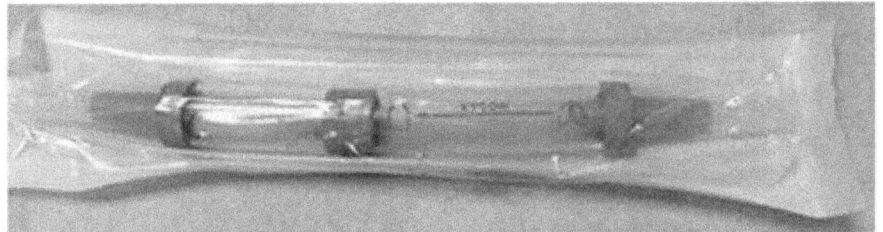

©A.M./N.L.

Think About It

• In neonatology and trauma, think the diagnosis of pneumothorax using the transillumination and/or ultrasound.

• During the installation of the one-way valve of type Heimlich: Pay attention to the direction of the valve (arrow on the device).

• Never leave a drain clamped long, if the latter does not drain, the pneumothorax risk of re-accumulate.

Memo 45

Electrocardiogram (ECG)

I ♦ positioning of electrodes

♦ position of limb lead electrodes
R for right : member upper right (red).
The for the left : member left upper (yellow).
N for neutral : member lower right (black).
Mnemonic: "the blood (red) on the bitumen (black), the sun (yellow) on the prairie (green)".
The roots (shoulders and iliac spines), least of parasites, no influence on the amplitude, but risk of change in axis, with appearance or disappearance of anomalies in 10% of cases.

♦ Position of Chest Leads
To place in this order++:
- **V1:** 4th intercostal space law - Edge of the sternum;
- **V2:** 4th intercostal space left - Edge of the sternum;
- **V4:** 5e intercostal space left - Mid-clavicular line;
- **V6:** horizontal even that V4 - axillary line average;
- **V3:** mid-distance between V2 and v4;
- **V5:** mid-distance between V4 and V6 anterior axillary line.

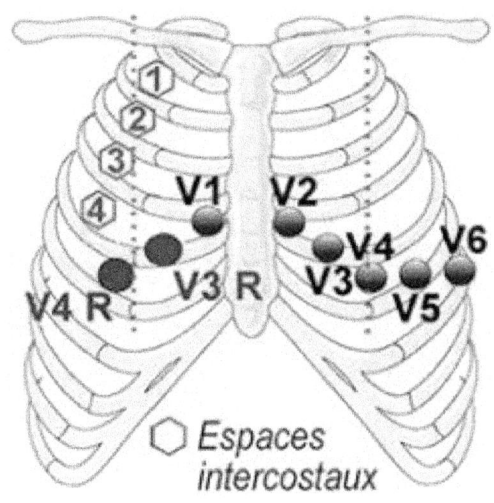

♦ **position of complementary electrodes**
- **V7 to V9:** horizontal even as V4, V5, V6;
- **V7:** posterior axillary line;
- **V8:** Tip of the scapula;
- **V9:** mid distance between V8 and the thorny after the spine;
- **V4R:** 5th intercostal space law - Mid-clavicular line;
- **V3R:** mid-distance between V1 and V4R.

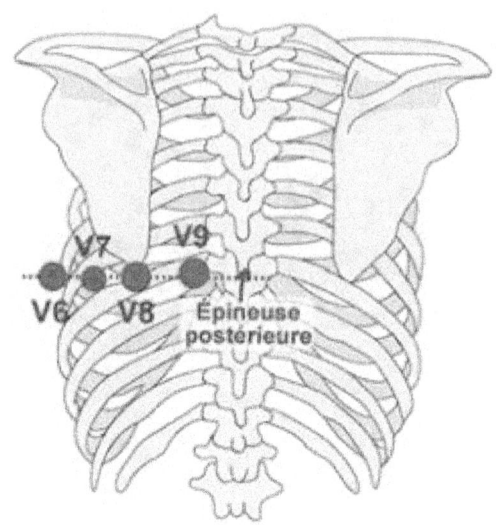

II Audit ♦

• Standard Settings:
- Speed for the conduct of the paper: 25 mm/s (1 Petit carreau = 0.04 s);
- Amplitude of registration: 10 mm/mV (1 Petit carreau = 0.01 mV);
- Filter for the reduction of parasites on "on".
• Leads all recorded?
• P wave in D1 positive? Otherwise check the position of the electrodes devices.
• Line of regular basis? If scrapie or anarchic, make sure of the rest of the patient.
Enter the identity of the patient or the note on the ECG, dial the ECGS++.

Memo 46
Transport Incubator

I ♦ Definition
The incubator, called familiarly "brooder", is a medical device reproducing to the maximum the fetal conditions, in order to maintain normothermia of the new-born and the premature.
There are several types of incubators:

- The incubator closed ;

- The incubator opened or radiant (double wall or simple wall according to the weight of the new-born);

- The incubator of transport.

The new-born is located in a zone of air heated pool, the loss of heat by convection are diminished, the losses by conductions are virtually nil thanks to the foam mattress. The hot air warms the walls which avoids the loss of heat by radiation.

II Technical ♦

♦ Hardware
Passenger compartment • in Plexiglas with 6 portholes (4 side doors and frontal 2). Accessibility of four sides which allows a comfort of intervention, the new-born remains in the heating part of the incubator during the gestures of resuscitation (the meaning of ventilation foot-allows head to maintain the temperature despite the opening of the portholes).
• Plateau of bedding (possibility of the Put in proclive, sometimes even to partially remove the incubator).

• Mattresses.

• Support the pipes fan.
• Thermal Probe skin. The incubators of transport do not have adjustment of the rate of moisture. In general the reduced time of transport limit the loss of water from the new-born.

• To the outside: TABLE command to adjust, to monitor the temperature of the new-born and the incubator (air mode = measured at the level of the mattress, and Skin Mode = temperature measured by the sensor to the skin).
• Connection sector and integrated battery.

♦ **settings**
Control mode selected by the user: the more often the regulating mode skin, the system module The heating in function of the skin temperature measured and that requested. Attention to the proper application of the probe on the skin of the newborn.

♦ **Maintenance**

• Cleaning between each patient :
- Put the incubator at the judgment;
- Clean the incubator once it is empty, if possible, wait until the temperature of the incubator or ambient temperature;
- Clean inside and outside the passenger compartment, the receiving party of the plateau, the plateau and the mattress to the help of products adapted (detergent disinfectant non-toxic validated by the direction of the establishment);
- Never use alcohol, ether, or grease.
• *Weekly cleaning* : each element of the incubator is removed to be cleaned separately.
• Trace the disinfections.

>>> Transport Incubator of type Médipréma®

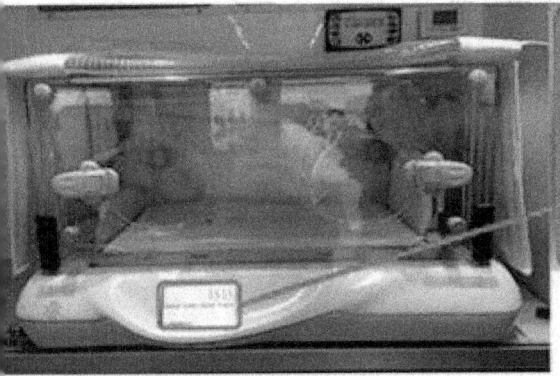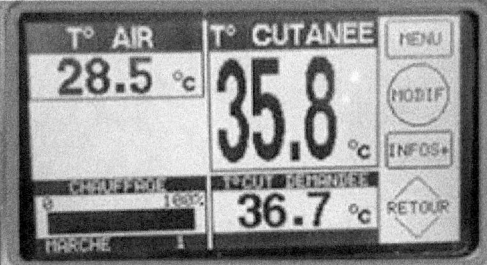

Affichage : programmation et surveillance de la température

©A.M./N.L.

Memo 47

Immobilization on a hard plan

I ♦ Definition

The plan hard with Head immobilizer is used to immobilize a victim suspicious of a trauma of the spinal column.
By immobilising the whole body of a victim, the plan allows hard to respect the axis head-neck-trunk and limit any onset or worsening of a possible lesion of the spinal column during the mobilization or the transport of the latter.

II Technical ♦

The ideal technique is that of the bearing in the soil of the victim to three teammates.

A crewmember placed behind the victim continues the maintenance of the head of the victim during the entire maneuver: it is he who guides and control the whole of the maneuver.

Another teammate place the hands of the victim on his thighs, and place the hard plan along the victim on the opposite side of the rollover.

Then the two teammates are placed in the knees on the side of the turning at the level of the chest and the basin of the victim. They seize the victim on the opposite side of the reversal at the level of the shoulder, of the basin and of the lower limbs that must remain aligned. They turn the victim to them: The rotation is done slowly and of a block, it is stopped as soon as the victim is on the side.

The other crew member accompanies the movement to keep the head in the axis of the trunk.

The two teammates slides the hard plan under the back of the victim until it Vienna is pressed against the victim and that the head cushion is well positioned at the level of the head.

When the hard plan is in place, they based the victim and the plan drive gently on the ground and mesh the head of the victim at the hard plan by placing successively the blocks side immobilisateurs on each side of the head and the strap of Frontal fixing then chin strap.

At the end of the maneuver, team members can then release the maintenance of the head and fasten the victim on the hard plan using a strap spider.

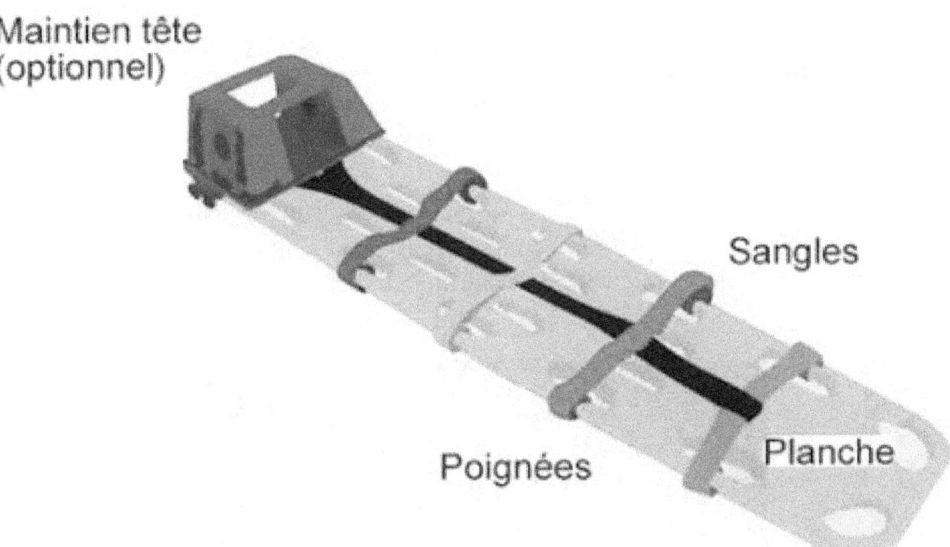

Maintien tête (optionnel)

Sangles

Poignées

Planche

© L.D.

Memo 48

Intubation

I ♦ Definition

The tracheal intubation is a technique in support of the Airways which is to insert a probe into the trachea.

II Technical ♦

♦ Choice of the blade

There are different types of laryngoscopes, blades to use unique or non-unique. The laryngoscope contains a handle and a straight blade or curve.

→ *for intubation of the new-born* : prefer straight blades (the anatomy of the upper airway is different of the Child and the adult, the glottal port is higher and earlier than in the adult):

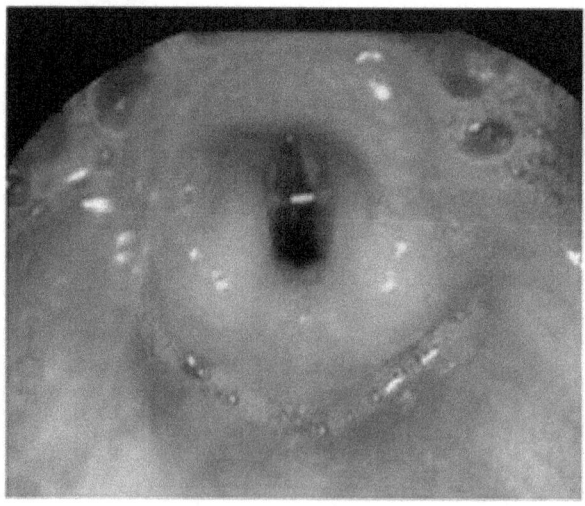

©A.M./N.L.

→ The choice of the size can be done by measuring with the blade the distance which goes from the lips of the child up to the larynx.

♦ **Choice of the probe**

There are several methods to choose the size of the probe to intubation.

For a child over two years, several formulas are used:

$$\left(\frac{\text{Âge} + 16}{4}\right) \pm 0{,}5^* = \text{Diamètre en millimètres de la sonde}$$

* - 0.5 in case of the use of probe of intubation to balloon.

Diameter of the Ear child = diameter of the probe of intubation (unreliable method)

Age	Weight	Size of probe	The Blades		
Premature	< 2-2.5 kg	2.5 mm	Miller 0-00		
New-born at term	2-3.5 kg	3 mm			
	≥ 3.5 kg	3.5 mm			
	2-6 months 4-8 kg		Miller 0-1	3.5 mm	Miller 1-Oxford-Mac 1
	6-12 months 8-12 kg			4 mm	Miller 1-Oxford-Mac 1

	12-18 months		4.5 mm	Miller 1-Oxford-Mac 1
	18-4 years		5 mm	Mac 2
	4 years		5.5 mm	Mac 2
	6 years		6 mm	Mac 2
	8 years		6.5 mm	Mac 3
	10 years		7 mm	Mac 3
	12 years		7.5 mm	Mac 3
	14 years		7.5-8 mm	Mac 3

→ In neonatology, probes of intubation to canaliculi are used to inject of surfactant in intra-tracheal.

→ To predict provision, when intubation, several different sizes (A probe more small and a probe greater than 0.5 mm).

→ Use of balloon catheter contraindicated in the new-born < 1 month (risk of stenosis), the narrowness of the cartilage cricoïde serves as a natural balloon.

>>> *The* probes of intubation to canalicule (left), without ballonet (middle) and with ballonet (right)

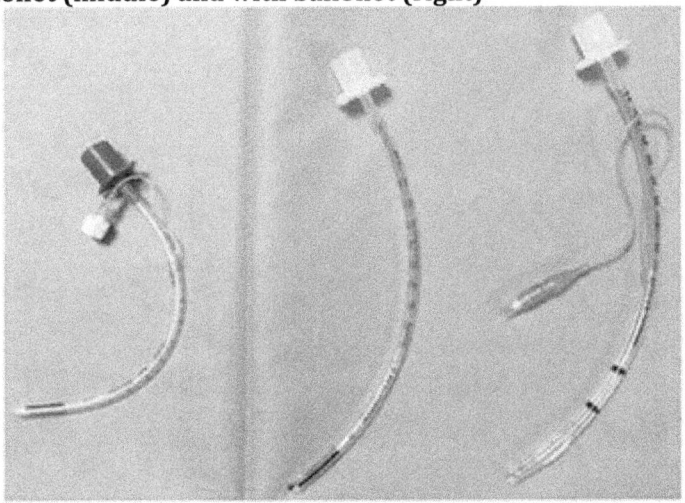

©A.M./N.L.

♦ **mark on the probe**
• In the new-born, prefer the nasotrachéale intubation. In case of emergency (very poor adaptation to the extrauterine life), intubation faster by oral route is justified.

Calculation of the mark on the probe visible at the edge or narinaire to the Dental arcade

New-born	• 7 + weight (by nasal)
	• 6 + weight (oral)

| Child | • To the nose: 15 + age in years / 2
• At the arcade Dental: 12 + age in years / 2
• Or: size of the probe × 3 |

- Check the correct positioning of the probe to the auscultation: Ventilation symmetrical. The measurement of the capnométrie confirms the good intratracheal position (see Mémo 39 Capnographie/Capnométrie).

♦ **Hardware of intubation**

- Mandrel if needed (can be used in the case of difficult intubation in the child, never in the newborn).
- Magill forceps (Sizes adapted).
- Sterile gloves.
- Vial of sterile water to lubricate the probe of intubation (neonatal, infant) or lubricants sterile (spray or gel).
- Syringe of 5 ml to inflate the balloon (the balloon is connected to a unidirectional valve on one of the sides of the sensor, its tank allows you to know if the latter is well inflated), use a specific gauge to inflate and monitor the pressure of the balloon in the second intension, the latter must be < 20 cmH2O.
- Union of Beaufils: allows a better oxygenation of the child during the intubation. Connected between the probe of intubation (size 2.5/3/3.5) and the fitting of Cobb, it brings the oxygen thanks to its connection to the respirator or the ball to one-way valve or to the T-piece.
- Hardware: adhesive tape (fibranne, woven, or tape ELASTOPLAST type®, if available cord for the greatest).

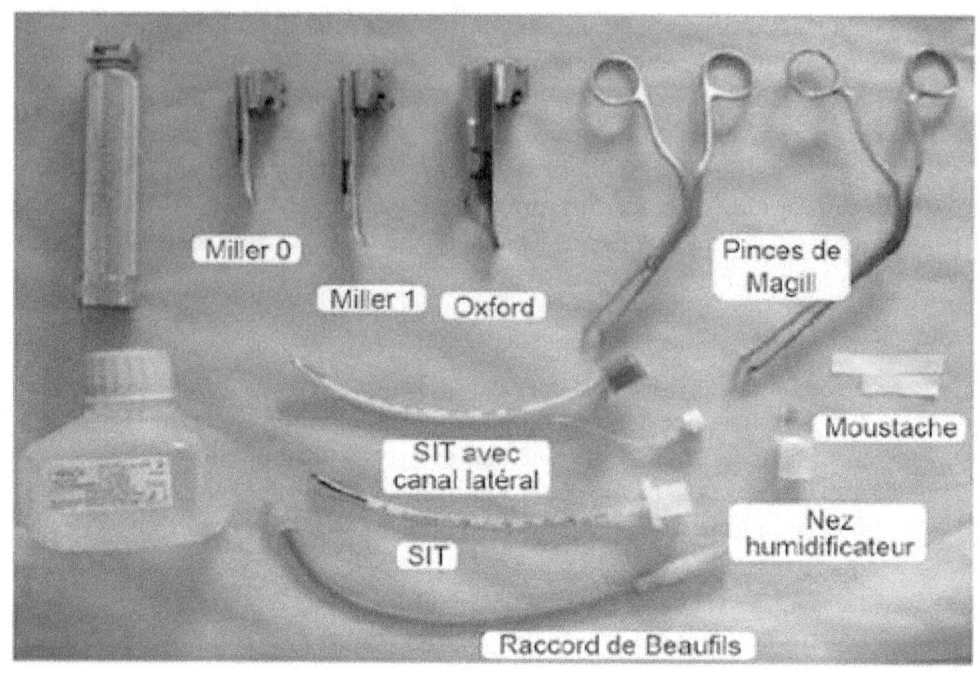

©A.M./N.L.

♦ fixing

>>> Positioning of the adhesive on the probe of intubation

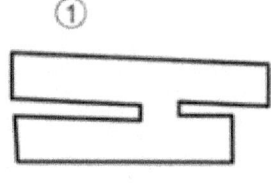 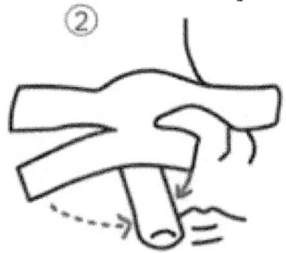 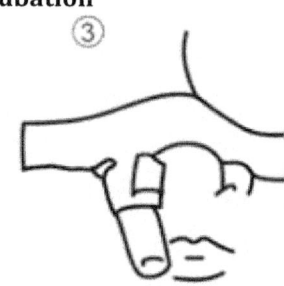

©A.M./N.L.

>>> fixing of the probe

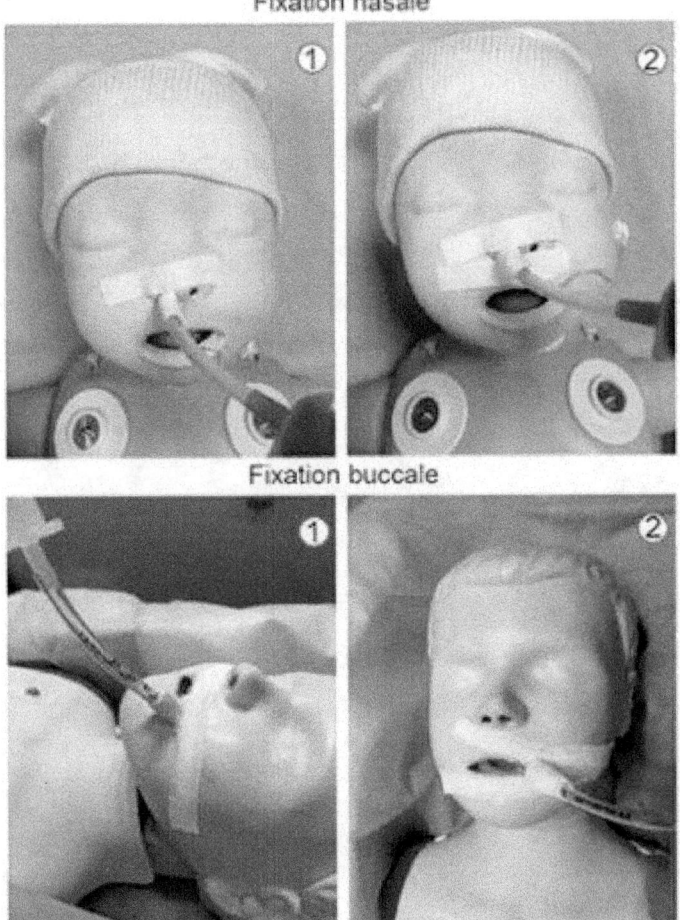

©A.M./N.L.

Think About It

• In the case of laryngoscope to blades not disposable, always provide the batteries and spare bulbs in the event of incorrect operation of the laryngoscope, the projected light must be white: if yellow, change the bulb.

• In the case of use of disposable blades, provide available a set of blades not disposable if difficult intubation.

• Equipment of aspiration ready and verified before the realisation of the gesture.

• Lung Auscultation symmetrical.

• Monitoring of expired CO_2.

• Equipment for difficult intubation: See Mémo 49.

Memo 49
Difficult intubation

I ♦ Definition
Intubation is a delicate gesture and a critical period in the support for the seriously ill child. Some anatomical and physiological characteristics in the newborn and the child can make the gesture of intubation more difficult for a practitioner less experienced in pediatrics. Some factors may be identified as predictors of a difficult intubation. However, even without any risk factor, a newborn child or a child may prove difficult to intubate her (the orifice glottal is higher and earlier than in the adult).

♦ Risk Factors for a difficult intubation
• Premature Large < 26 SA.
• Congenital Malformations affecting the airway, the region craniofaciale cervical or (for example: syndrome of Pierre-Robin, cleft palate, disease of overload, trisomy 21, syndrome of Crouzon, etc.).
• Facial trauma.
• Multiple trauma (cervical column immobilized).
• Obstruction of the upper airway (foreign body, severe laryngitis, anaphylaxis, etc.).
• Subglottic Stenosis.
• Tonsillar hypertrophy (the suspect in the child with a night hum).
→ at any time, when a team is faced with a difficult intubation, it is lawful to ask the reinforcement of a paediatric team, another team or a particular hardware.

II Technical ♦

♦ Hardware
Intubation is a gesture that request a minimum of preparation.
• Balloon to one-way valve (BAVU), or device of the workpiece in the T for a new-born, with a mask of appropriate size.
• Vacuum Cleaner of mucus.

• Source of oxygen or a mixture air/O2 for a new-born.
→ The hardware of intubation is chosen according to the size and weight of the child.
→ In case of difficult intubation, specific equipment must be easy to access and the team must know the use.

This situation is rare, it is good to train regularly to its use.

Technical ♦
• *The positioning of the new-born or of the child is extremely important* to optimize the chances of success. In the case of difficult intubation, the position of the patient is reviewed before to perform a new attempt. In the new-born, the common error is to perform a hyperextension of the neck, there is the need to keep a neutral position of the head and in the older child put possibly the head in slight extension with a log under the shoulders. The position of the operator, sometimes precarious in pre-hospital care, is optimized (height of the patient, release the space, etc.).
• For intubation tracheal NASO of new-born *in the case of difficult passage of the posterior nares, do not force, introduce a small probe of the suction or gastric in the nostril once the choana crossed, slide the probe of intubation by above.*
• *In the case of difficult visualization of the vocal cords in the young child, by reason of a epiglottis anatomically generous, the use of a straight blade helps to see the glottis. A blade of Oxford (see* Mémo 48 Intubation) is often useful to improve the visualization in the infant or the new-born at term and helps to identify the language. In the premature < 28 Its some blades 00 are a little wider than others, do not hesitate to change equipment for better exposure.
• A pressure on the cartilage cricoïde can sometimes help the visualization. The latter must not be too large because this could prevent the insertion of the probe.
• After crossing of vocal cords, *in case of the stop of the probe on the anterior wall of the trachea, we can be led to deflect the head of the premature.*
• *In case of nasal intubation, the Magill forceps is used when the visualization of the glottis is adequate to guide the probe between the vocal cords in remaining to 2 cm from the end of the probe. In the*

case of oral intubation, it is rarely useful, a rotation movement may suffice.
- It is possible to adapt a fitting of Beaufils between the end of the probe and the Bavu, or part in t, to oxygenate the new-born during intubation (see Mémo 48).
- A patient can be difficult to intubate her, but relatively easy to ventilate the Bavu.

- In the case of difficult ventilation at the Bavu, you can try:
- To break down to 2 operators: one holds the mask to improve the sealing, the other compresses the flask slowly;
- To use an oropharyngeal airway;
- Ask a second operator to luxer the lower jaw forward.
- The patient must always be resumed at the Bavu or with the device of the workpiece in the T between the tests of intubation. A gastric distension occurs quickly and impedes the ventilation, a gastric tube is asked to empty the stomach.
- In the infant and child, it is possible to use a mandrel of Eschmann, or equivalent, on which you can insert in advance a probe of intubation lubricated (gel, spray or sterile water).
- *In the case of the crossing of the glottis and the impossibility of passage of the probe, suspect a stenosis under glottal (patient with history of intubation or congenital stenosis), thinking to resort to a probe of lower caliber.*

If, despite these techniques, intubation remains impossible, other methods exist:
- Laryngeal Mask: soft mask inserted in the blind in the pharynx. The size of the device must be selected depending on the size of the patient. The device is attached after the insertion and its monitored position, because it can move during transportation. This device is very little used in neonatology, except in operating block for certain malformations, and only for a weight > 2 kg.
- Vidéolaryngoscope: several devices allow to maximize the visualization of the glottal space, some do not have the equivalent of the small sizes of conventional laryngoscopes and are not

suitable for new-born babies and infants, and none should be for premature infants.
• Retrograde intubation with technique of Seldinger.
• Cricothyroïdotomie to the needle or with a device of percutaneous cricothyroïdotomie (see Mémo 42).
• *In case of failure of intubation but an adequate ventilation to the Bavu, a transport of short duration with a ventilation at the Bavu can be envisaged. Intubation will be retried in hospital with access to additional resources and staff. The team in préhospitalier will notify the service receiver of the situation so that the staff prepares to welcome this type of patient and is already mobilizing the necessary resources.*

>>> **Vidéolaryngoscopes (left), MC graft® (middle) and masks laryngés (right)**

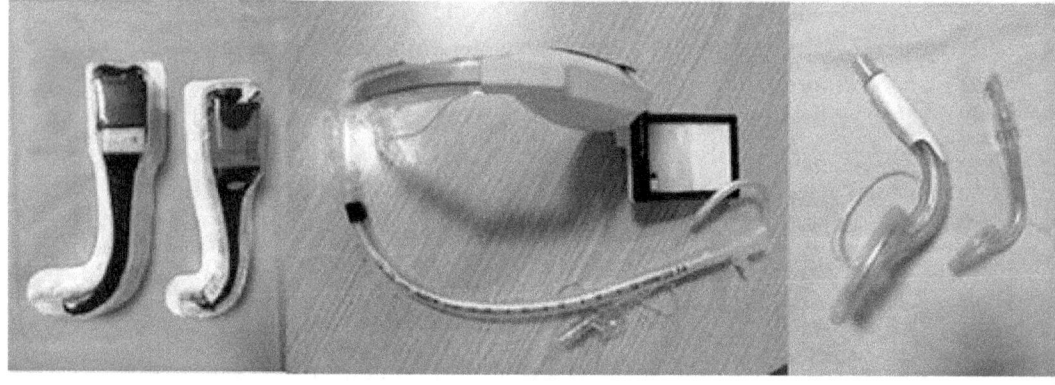

©A.M./N.L.

>>> **Laryngeal Mask**

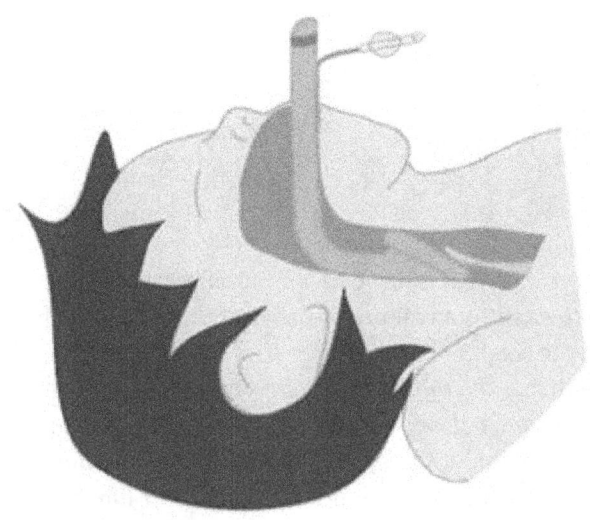

Think About It

• Except in the case of ACR, sedation-analgesia is carried out. If the latter is inadequate at the first attempt, it is optimized before a new test.

• Monitoring.

• The FASTRACH® is only usable in the child of more than 30 kg.

Memo 50

Vacuum mattress (MID)

I ♦ Definition

The *vacuum mattress* is used to immobilise the whole body of a victim suspected of a trauma of the head, the spinal column, basin and/or of the thigh.

By immobilising the whole body of a victim, the MID allows you to respect its axis head-neck-trunk and limit any onset or worsening of a possible lesion of the spinal column during the mobilization or transport. It also allows to immobilise the lower limbs.

II Technical ♦

The installation of a victim on the MID is performed using a technique to lift the bridge.

Place the mid in the vicinity of the victim in a suitable position to the technique of hitch used.

Open the valve to allow the entry of the air and distribute the balls.

Stiffen moderately the MID falling within the sides to facilitate the maneuver, put in place a cloth or a coverage of survival.

Once the victim filed on the MID, put in form the mattress around his body: for this, closer to the edges of the mattress of hand and on the other of the head of the victim, maintain the side edges of the Mattress along the victim without the mobilize with the help of the retaining straps, and then make the vacuum inside the mattress in sucking air with a suction device until the mattress becomes hard. Close the valve and disconnect the suction device, and finally adjust the retaining straps.

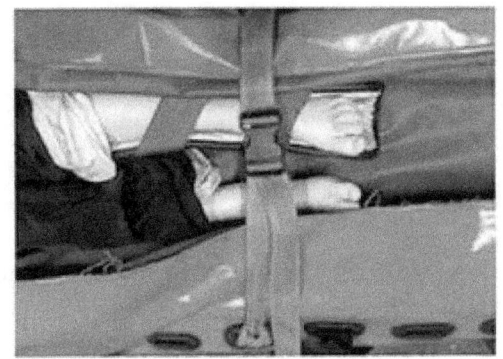

© L.D.

Memo 51
Oxygen Therapy

I ♦ Definition
Material of passive oxygenation used in the infant and the child with a spontaneous breathing effective.

II Technical ♦

♦ nasal glasses
System of oxygenation at low flow rate (between 0.25 l to 4 l/min of O2) which delivers to a maximum of 35 % of oxygen.
• Beyond 4 l/min, oxygen must be warmed and humidified.
• The glasses are placed in the nostrils of the child.
• There are several sizes adapted (Premature, new-born, pediatric, adult).

♦ Simple face mask
Plastic tank positioned on the mouth and the nose of the child.
• The air inspired and expired passes through the holes in each side.
• The mask remains in position thanks to an elastic positioned behind the head of the Child (several sizes ranging from infants to adults).
• The flow of oxygen must be a minimum of 6 l/min to evacuate the expired carbon dioxide.
• Oxygen Concentration of 40% to 60%.

♦ mask to high concentration
Simple mask equipped with a manifold tank of oxygen.
• The minimum flow rate must be 6 l/min.
• Fill the tank of the mask before the position on the face of the Child, the tank must remain inflated during the inspiration and expiration, if this is not the case, adapt the oxygen flow (pediatric size and adult).
• Allows you to reach up to 97% of oxygen concentration.

♦ **nebulizer mask**
System of oxygenation and nebulisation. It is a simple mask equipped with a receptacle for the nebulization of certain treatments (size ranging from infants to adults).

>>> devices of oxygen therapy

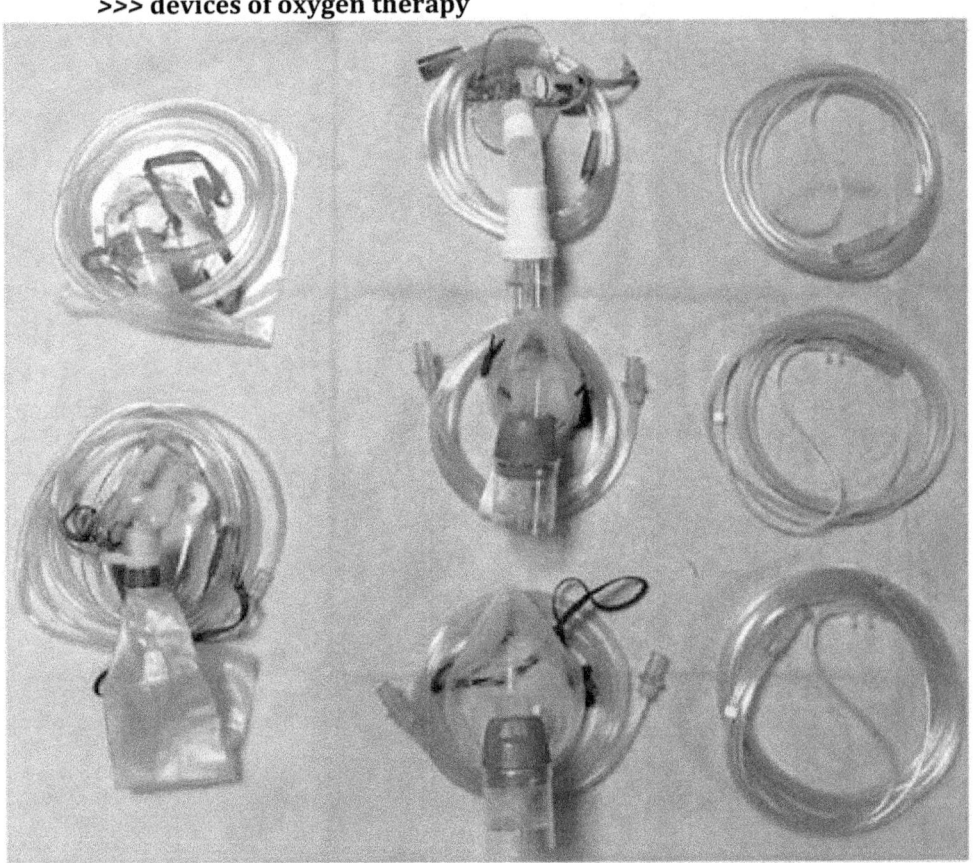

Masque à haute concentration   Masque nébuliseur   Lunettes à oxygène

© A.M./N.L.
Think About It

- Use of the humidified oxygen to the extent possible, humidification prevents the drying of the mucous membranes.
- A flow rate high in relation to the weight of the child brings a positive end expiratory pressure (PEP), which is not quantified: 2 l/kg/min ≈ +4 cmH2O. This PEP is variable according to the child, the diameter of the nostril, leaks...

Memo 52

Lateral position of Security (PLS)

I ♦ Definition
Any unconscious victim who breathes, or sleepy, must be placed on the side in *lateral position of security.*
The PLS allows to maintain the freedom of the upper airway because it prevents the fall of the language back and it limits the footprint by allowing the liquid to flow to the outside of the mouth kept open.

II Technical ♦
• Remove the glasses of the victim if it to door.
• Ensure that its members below are elongated coast to coast. If this is not the case, the gently closer to one another, in the axis of the body of the victim.
• Place the arm of the victim, the closest to the side of the flipper, at right angles to its body, then bend his elbow while keeping the palm of his hand turned toward the top. The alignment of the legs and the position of the upper member anticipate the final position.
• Move to knees or in tripod to the side of the victim.
A hand, enter the opposite arm of the victim, place the back of his hand against his ear, side first-aider.
Maintain the hand of the victim pressed against his ear, Palm against palm. During the rollover, the maintenance of the hand of the victim against his ear allows you to accompany the movement of the head and to decrease the bending of the cervical column that could aggravate a possible trauma.
With the other hand, catch the opposite leg, just behind the knee, the raise while keeping the foot to the ground.
• Move far enough away from the victim, at the level of the chest, to be able to turn to the side without having to back away.
Pull on the leg in order to roll the victim to the rescuer until the knee touches the ground.

Gently disengage the hand of the first aider who is placed under the head of the victim. To do this, and to avoid any mobilization of the head of the victim, maintain the elbow of the victim with the hand that held the knee.

Adjust the leg, located above, so that the hip and knee are at a right angle. The position of the leg from the top of the victim allows you to stabilize the PLS.

• Open the mouth of the victim with the thumb and the index finger of one hand without mobilizing the head, in order to allow the flow of fluids to the outside, and check that the position of the head preserves efficient ventilation.

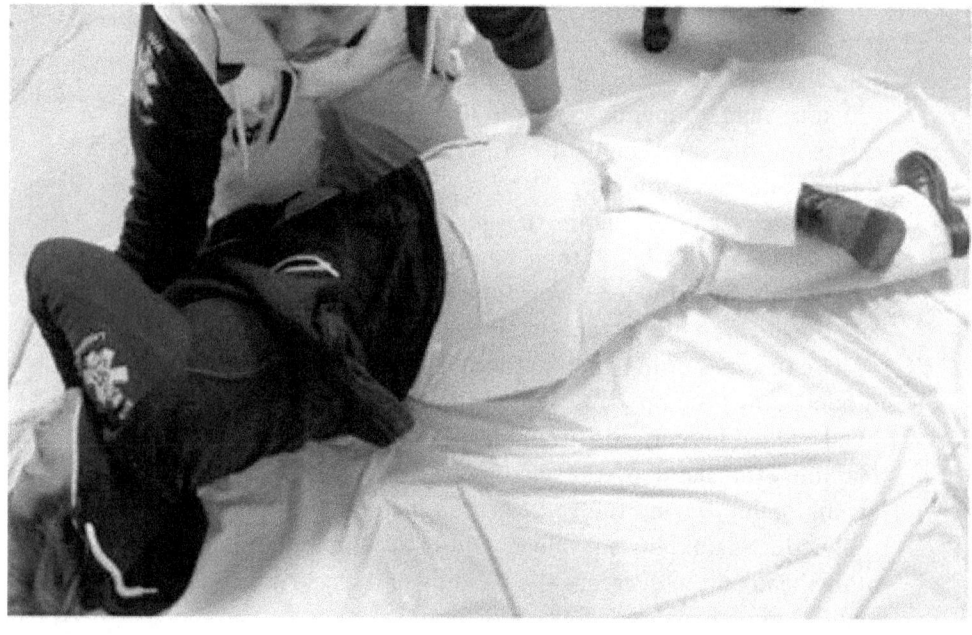

© L.D.

Think About It

- A *pregnant woman* or an *overweight child* will be put in PLS on the left side to avoid the compression of certain vessels of the abdomen.
- The development in PLS involves certain risks in the *traumatized of the vertebral column, in particular neck. That is why it is preferable to conduct the technique to at least two teammates and put in place a cervical collar on the victim before its rollover.*

Memo 53
Procedures for radiotelephony

I ♦ the call
• Always set out the indicative of the post that you call, then do follow the your (e.g. : " SAMU of the UMH... ").
• Always ensure that no communication is in progress.
• Limit the communication to the essential in speaking clearly.

♦ *The* force of signals
• Fort/strong enough/Low/very low.

♦ Legibility of signals
Clear/readable/distorted/with interference/Unreadable/inaudible (e.g. : " I receive you loud and clear ").

II ♦ conventional expressions
• *The* affirmative = "Yes".
• Negative = "No".
• Answer = "My transmission is ended and I expect a response on your part."
• Stand-by = "wait until I remind you".
• Repeat = "repeat your last transmission or the specified part".
• Completed = "This transmission is complete and I do not expect a response".
• I listen = "pass your message".
• Collationnez = "Repeat All this message, or the specified part, exactly as you have received".
• Correction = "An error has been committed in this message, the correct text is... ".
• Correct = "C is correct".
• Confirm = "confirm me that you have well received... or confirm to me that I have understood... ".
• How do you receive? = " What is the readability of my transmission? ".

III ♦ spelling of letters

The international alphabet is used to spell the names clean, the important words or confusing: it prevents before specifying " I spelled ". For a letter doubled, it is said " twice ".

A = Alfa	N = November
B = Bravo	O = Oscar
C = Charlie	P = Papa
D = Delta	Q = Quebec
E = Echo	R = Romeo
F = Foxtrot	S = Sierra
G = Golf	T = Tango
H = Hotel	U = Uniform
I = India	V = Victor
J = JULIETT	W = Whiskey
K = kilo	X = X-ray
The = Lima	Y = Yankee
M = Mike	Z = Zulu

IV ♦ Transmission of Numbers

0 = Zero: " I spelled: zero as nothing ".

1 = Unit: " I spelled: A all alone ."

2 = Two: " I spelled: A and A ".

3 = Three: " I spelled: two and a ".

4 = Four: " I spelled: two times two ."

5 = *five:* " *I spelled: Three and Two* ".

6 = *Six:* " *I spelled: two times three* ".

7 = *Seven:* " *I spelled: four and three* ".

8 = *eight:* " *I spelled: Two times four* ".

9 = *nine:* " *I spelled: five and four* ".
Decimal point: "decimal place".

A number is transmitted by utterance of each of the figures that the consist of:

- 10 = unit zero;
- 125 = Unit two five;
- 1 230 = Unit TWO THREE ZERO.

Memo 54

Hitch to three teammates and four teammates

I ♦ hitch to three teammates

♦ Definition

The techniques of raise a victim to three teammates are carried out if the victim is not suspicious of a trauma of the spinal column.
These techniques allow to install a victim on a stretcher.

Technical ♦

Dutch bridge to three teammates: a teammate, placed in a bridge above the head of the victim guide and in overall command of the maneuver.
Another crew member is placed in a bridge above the feet of the victim, the last team member is placed in a bridge above the victim between the other two.
Have the stretcher along the body of the victim, reduce its before-arm on its trunk.
Two teammates must be facing, take a position at the level of the feet and the head of the victim, the third crewmember must rely on the shoulder of the second to climb over the victim and ask his foot on the middle of the outer skirt of the stretcher.
The first teammate slides one hand under the back of the neck of the victim and the other under its shoulder blades, the second crewmember captures the dowels of the victim and the third commits its hands under the size of the victim and enters the side parts of the belt or the pants.
The team members should raise in keeping the back flat, raise the victim and the move laterally until the stretcher. The crewmember of head directs to ask the victim on the stretcher at the end of travel.

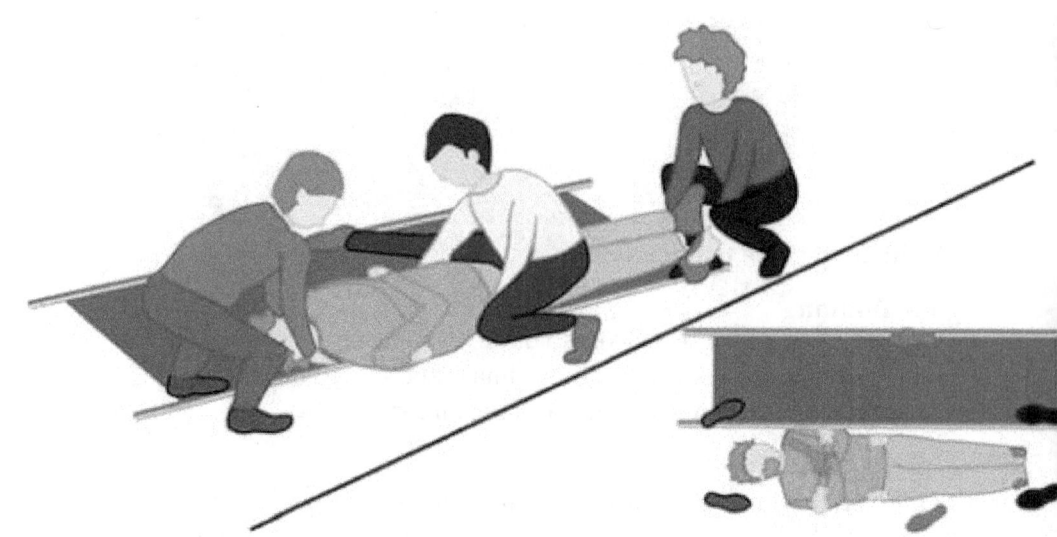

II ♦ Linkage to four teammates

♦ Definition

The techniques of raise a victim to four teammates are conducted if the victim is suspicious of a trauma of the spinal column.

Technical ♦

Dutch Bridge to Four teammates: the crewmember placed at the head of the victim in the ensures the maintenance by a Socket latéro-SIDE-TO-SIDE. It is positioned a knee stretcher side to earth, to the interior of the two stalks. It is he who guides and control the whole of the maneuver.

The fourth crewmember therefore keeping the head of the victim during the entire maneuver.

The rest of the technique is similar to the Dutch bridge to three teammates.

Memo 55

Monitoring during the transport

I ♦ Definition

Complications and a worsening of the condition of the patient can occur during transport. The security and the monitoring of the patient are under the responsibility of the team of the EMS.

Outside of a few rare cases: the great principle of transport pediatric is a stabilization before transport.

II Technical ♦

A. Before the transport (intervention Primary and Secondary)

• Note the constants of the patient at the departure of the supported to rely on reference values.
• Monitoring of infusions (nature, dilution, quantity for the transport, flow, labelling).
• Ensure the permeability of the venous track (swelling, redness, mounting).
• Ensure the correct mounting of different Probes and drains and note the marks (especially the probe of intubation: Check the pressure of the balloon with the pressure gauge (Always less than 20 cmH2O), check that the "whisker" fixing of adhere properly to the skin otherwise the repeat).
• Install the hardware in a manner that is accessible for the transportation: monitoring devices, rickshaw-syringes, respirator, drains, Bavu, vacuum cleaner to mucosities, venous track (identification of a track of emergency if you need to inject treatments during transport).
• Installation of the patient on the stretcher for the transfer: secure the equipment and the patient.
• Setting the Alarms for the transport (alarm high and low volume +), they will be adapted to the patients and therapeutic goals (see Mémo 1 Scores et constantes): scope (frequency cardiac and respiratory in function of the age, Saturation*, blood

pressure, apneas) TcPO2/TcPCO2 or expired CO2 (see Mémo 39 Capnographie/Capnométrie), fan (leaks, pressure high or low, FiO2, etc.) and alarm of the Incubator (temperature air and dermal).

* Monitoring of SpO2 with pre Setting the Alarms

New-born > 32 Its: 92% ≤ SpO2 ≤ 95%.

Large premature ≤ 32 Its: 87% < SpO2 ≤ 92%.

(Recommendations SFN 2016)

♦ **specific monitoring to the secondary transport or reinforcement of a team**
• Take knowledge of oral transmissions and written (verification of the contents of the file transfer: authorization of care, patient transfusion...).
• Keep only what is essential (empty the different pockets of collection, note the quantities, remove the pockets of empty infusion).
• Before leaving the service, remember to check the presence of two tie bands of identity on the child.

B. During Transport

• *Hemodynamic Monitoring* : note at regular intervals (depending on the stability of the patient and the time of transport) the oxygen saturation, blood pressure (program the automatic mode with an interval in adequacy with the status of the patient), heart rate, respiratory rate, the expired CO2 if the patient is intubated-ventilated, TcPO2/TcPCO2 (if it is a new-born or an infant in NIV or ventilation invasive), temperature, blood glucose capillary (if indicated by the pathology of the child).
• *Monitoring of ventilatory parameters* : check the settings programd ventilatory and note the measures of the respirator as the pressure of peak, the pressure of plateau, the inspiratory pressure, the PEP, the average pressure, the FiO2 ; monitor the percentage of leaks.
• *Clinical Surveillance* : Monitor the coloration of the patient (pallor, cyanosis), the onset or worsening of signs of a struggle, lung

auscultation to each mobilization of the patient, ensure its comfort and its security (good installation, Blanket, sheets, straps of the mattress-shell attached), monitoring of content (quantitative and qualitative) of different pockets of Collection: diuresis, drains, gastric probe.
• *Monitoring of infusions* : monitor the site of injection, keep an access to the track first of emergency, keep a visibility on the flow rates of the rickshaw-syringes and on the labelling of the syringes of infusion, ensure that the pipes are not cubits.
• *Evaluation of the Pain* : Rate the pain of the patient before the supported, during and at the end (EVENDOL, EVA, other scales of pain adapted to the age and the types of pain, chronic, acute, post-op...), note the signs of pain, discomfort, anxiety.

Think About It

• Fill in a sheet of monitoring nurse Medical and during transport. These sheets are duplicated, one is kept and archived, the other is handed over to the service in which is allowed the child. Perform oral transmissions and written, note all special events and treatments injected during the transport.

• In pediatrics, a special place will be made to the parents, to reassure them, their explain the conduct of the supported and transport, especially if they cannot accompany the child.

• Use of the means of distraction (games, lint, songs) to appease the child during the transfer (Unknown location, medical staff), use the parents as resource persons, ask them if the child has a Doudou and take knowledge of its centers of interest.

• The hypnoanalgésie is a method of increasingly widespread and used in préhospitalier, notably pediatrics to take in charge the anxiety and pain of the Child (in association with drug means).

Memo 56

Ventilation at the MASK

I ♦ Definition

Method of ventilation in intermittent positive pressure used in the infant and the child having a breath ineffective.

II Technical ♦

A. Ball to one-way valve (BAVU)

It can be connected to a source of oxygen. The one-way valve allows the evacuation of the expired air.

Hardware:

• The balloon must have a capacity of at least 450 ml for children and for new-born at term. In the absence of manual insufflator pressure controlled with T-piece, use a flask of 250 ml for premature babies.
• Masks (several sizes).
• Relief Valve (limited in most of the models to 40 cmH2O).
• Valve for Positive End Expiratory Pressure (PEEP) recommended for new-born babies.
• Oxygen Tank attached to the balloon, increases the oxygen concentration.
• Tubing with oxygen.
• Pressure Gauge recommended for new-born babies.

>>> BAVU With Pressure Gauge

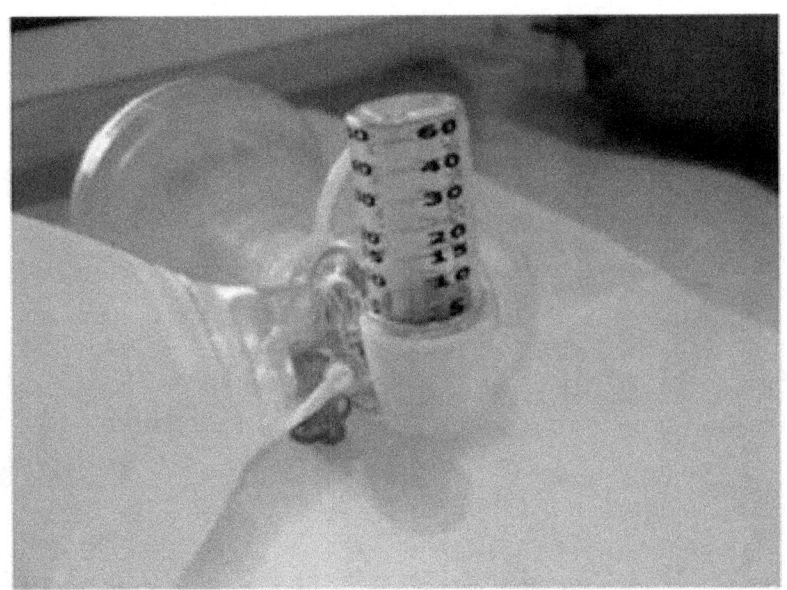

© A.M./N.L.

♦ newborns/infants
BAVU child model body weight < 15 kg.
Circular Mask to flexible edges in silicone (reduces the dead space): It must cover the root of the nose in the fold of the Chin without cover the eyes.
Technical: Head in a neutral position (the hyper-extension of the neck increases the airway obstruction), two fingers lifting the mandible without compressing the tissue under-mentonniers, apply the mask on the nose and the mouth open in order to allow a sealed application of the mask, making repeated cuts from the balloon to two fingers.

♦ Big Child
BAVU child body weight < 15 kg, adult BAVU weight > 15 kg.
Preformed Mask, it must cover the root of the nose in the fold of the Chin without cover the eyes.

Technical: > 2 years: Apply a slight extension of the neck (if no notion of trauma). Gently press the ball, as soon as the Chest raises release the pressure.

>>> BAVU Adult and Pediatric

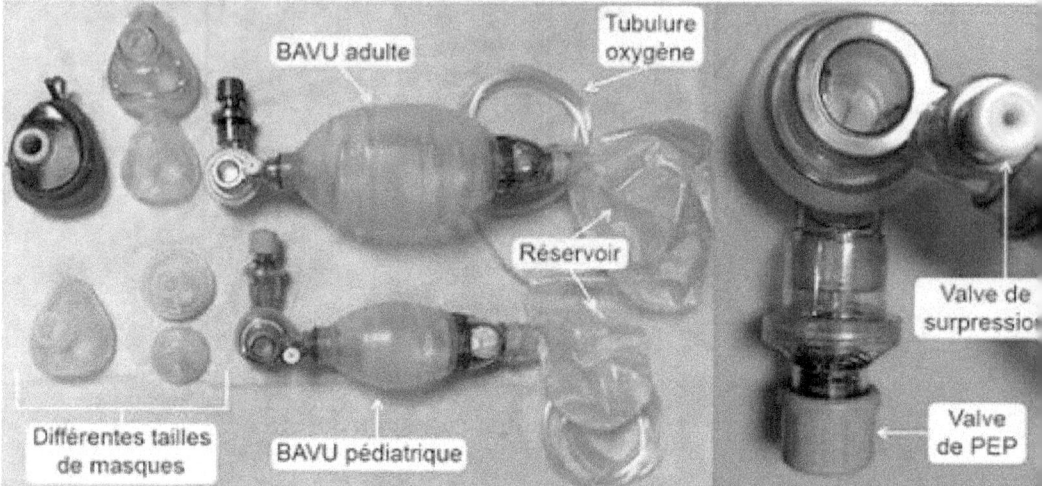

© A.M./N.L.

B. Device for T-piece of type NÉOPUFF®

Manual Fan, connected to a pressure gauge to check the insufflation pressure and adjust a PEP reliable. Thanks to this method the pressure and the time insufflation are more precise. It is used in the premature and the new-born at term.

The device of the workpiece in the type T NÉOPUFF® is connected to a source of oxygen, or to a mixer oxygen/air. The mask connected to the T-piece is swept by the oxygen/air mixture to the flow rate of the FiO2 set (for that the NÉOPUFF® correctly fitted its pressures, there must be a arrival of 10 l/min of MIXING O2/Air), an important advantage compared to the Bavu where no gas flows if we do not ballonne.

>>> manual insufflator pressure controlled with T-piece

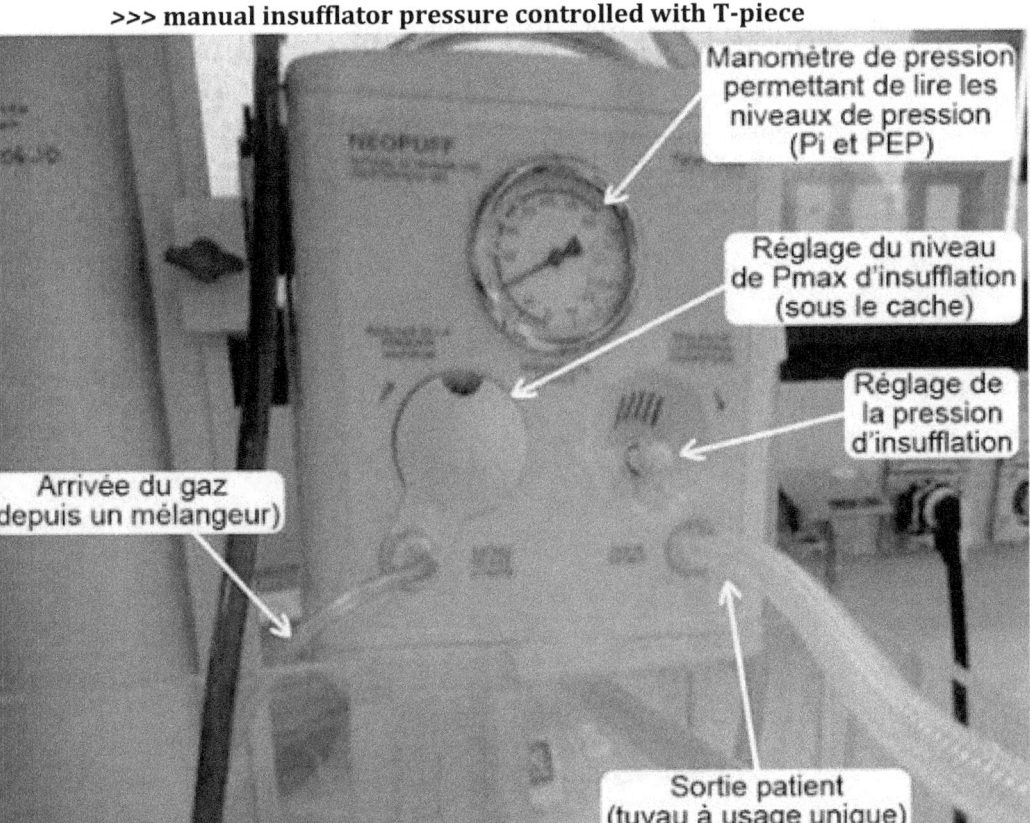

© A.M./N.L.

♦ **Hardware**
- *Device for T-piece of type NÉOPUFF®* composed of a pressure gauge (inspiratory pressure - PI - and PEP), an arrival of gas and an output patient.
- Pipe connected to the Mixer oxygen-air.
- Pipe connected to the Mask ranging to the child.
- Mask of suitable size.

Technical ♦

- The PEP must be set between 4-5 cmH2O, the adjustment is made at the level of the trackwheel fixed on the mask.

>>> Trackwheel PEEP valve

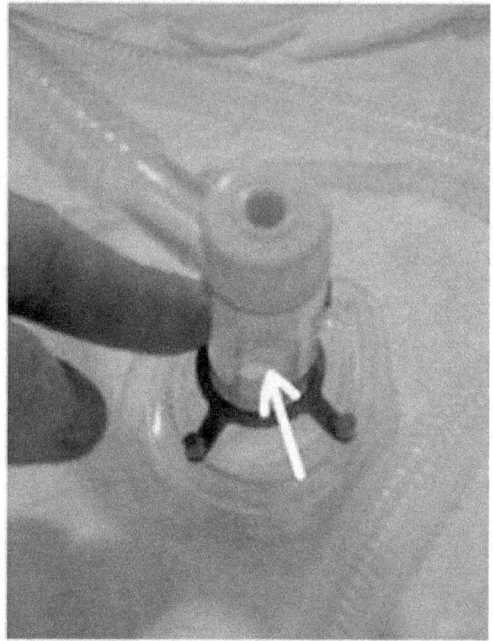

© A.M./N.L.
- The IP must be set:
- New-born at term: 20-25 cmH2O;
- Premature: 15-20 cmH2O.
- Maintain a hand the mask on the nose and the mouth of the new-born, enabling a good sealing, head in a neutral position.
- Breathe by plugging the hole of the valve, inspiratory with a finger of the hand holding the mask.

>>> insufflation by plugging the hole of the valve inspiratory

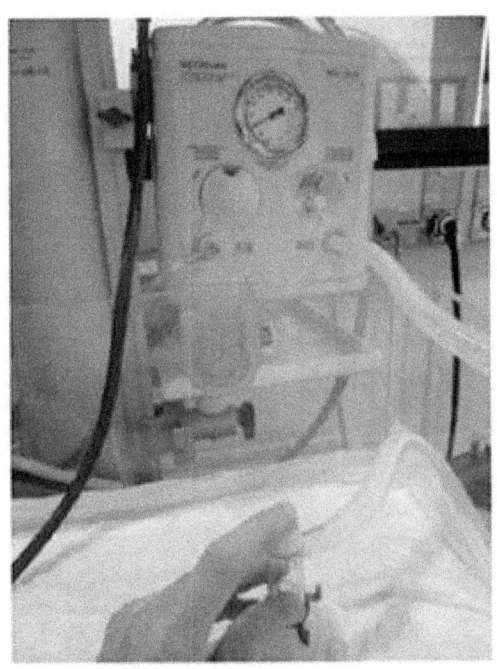

© A.M./N.L.
• For each ventilation, the needle of the gauge should rise up to the PI chosen and walk down to the level of the PEP SET.
• Monitor the oxygen according to the saturation of the new-born.

Think About It

• Excessive ventilation is harmful (volume, pressure and frequency).

• The manual ventilation in positive pressure can cause a gastric distension, think to ask a gastric tube to decompress the stomach.

Reminder of the oxygen saturation measured in susductale (right hand) in the first 10 minutes of life:

The values SpO2 acceptable after the birth	
2 minutes	60%
3 minutes	70%
4 minutes	80%
5 minutes	85%
10 minutes	90%

Memo 57

Mechanical ventilation

I ♦ Definition
This technique is to use a device for respiratory assistance, in order to supplement or attend the spontaneous ventilation of a patient intubated.

II Technical ♦

A. Conventional ventilation: new-born and small infants
• Fan Type " carver of Flux" sensor with proximal spirometry. The respirators former without synchronization are to be avoided.
• Pressure controlled (barometric mode), volume variable current according to the resistances of the airway, circuit, of changes in compliance and leaks around the probe of intubation.
• Continuous Flow.
• Inspiratory Time defined.
• Synchronization (trigger) - Synchronization of the beginning of the inspiration:
- To some spontaneous cycles (SIMV mode);
- Or to all spontaneous cycles (mode VAC);
- By adapting the inspiratory time (TI) at Ti useful: the time when the inspiratory flow decreases to a set value (Mode I);
- By regulating the pressure to deliver a controlled volume or a volume guaranteed (mode VG, not present on all brands of respirator).

♦ Modes
• *Synchronized intermittent mandatory ventilation (SIMV)* : recommended mode for new-born babies. The trigger can only be triggered a number of times, the frequency is controlled and secured. The flow of the inspiratory cycle of the respirator is synchronized with the cycle of the new-born. Between the cycles of the respirator, the new-born can trigger spontaneous cycles.

• *Assisted ventilation controlled (VAC)* : The spontaneous cycles of the new-born are assisted by the respirator, the inspiratory pressure and the duration of the inspiratory time are laid down.

♦ **settings**
• *Inspiratory fraction in O2* : FiO2 according to SpO2, sensor positioned to the right hand in the first hours of life (SUS values ductales) and PO2/TCPCO2 the skin electrodes on the chest.
• *Pressure settings of the pressure* : inspiratory pressure (Pi) = 16 to 20 cmH2O (the lowest possible). Positive End Expiratory Pressure (PEEP) = + 4 cmH2O The more often. Do not hesitate to take a specialized opinion.
• *The time parameters* : inspiratory time (Ti) = 0.3-0.4 (< 0.4 especially if premature < 33 weeks of aménorrhées) and expiratory time (te) long (I/E close to 1/2).

Attention: If Ti too long = Expiry active against a PI imposed = barotrauma and if te too short = auto-PEP.
• *Flow rate machine* : 8-12 l/min depending on the respirators.
• *Frequency* : 40 to 60/min (I/E ≈ 1/2).

• Inspiratory trigger the more sensitive possible.
→ on some devices, enable the volume guaranteed (no consensus of Neonatologists).

♦ **Monitoring of the spirometry spirometry**
• Current Volume (Vτ) = 5 to 7 ml/kg (before surfactant) not adjusted. A proximal sensor allows you to assess the synchronization between the child and the respirator, measure the values spirometric not settled in the child.
• A level of high leakage in a patient with a serious requiring the use of ventilatory parameters High leads to the réintuber with a probe of a half additional caliber.
• Monitoring of the FiO2 is mandatory on all neonatal respirators.
• The settings are to adapt according to the term and the pathology and to change very quickly after instillation of surfactant and according to the improvement of the clinical (SpO2/TCPCO2

the skin: see Mémo 39 Capnographie/Capnométrie and Mémo 55 Surveillance pendant le transport).

B. Conventional ventilation: Child
The fans identical to the adult models, respirators to intermittent flow.

♦ **Modes**
• Ventilation volume controlled (VVC): The current volume is set and the pressure is variable.
• Breakdown in controlled pressure (VPC): The pressure is set and the current volume is variable.
• Ventilation with inspiratory assistance (AI): When the patient begins an inspiration This triggers the fan, it sends an inspiratory flow high which minimizes the inspiratory effort of the patient.

♦ **settings**
• *Current Volume* (Volume instilled to the patient each cycle: VT: 6-8 ml/kg).

• Respiratory frequency.

• Report I/E.

• Maximum Pressure (P max).

• Positive End Expiratory Pressure (PEEP).
• *Inspiratory Trigger in flow* (the more sensitive as possible, without auto-triggering).

C. Ventilation at high frequency (HFO)
Indications: failure of the conventional ventilation, dysplasia broncho-pulmonary, hypercapnia and refractory hypoxemia, congenital diaphragmatic hernia, acute respiratory distress syndrome (ARDS).
This breakdown combines the ventilatory frequency high and laid down (> 300 cycles per minute) and a small current volume, lower than the dead space. The oscillation generated by a piston or a diaphragm creates vibrations in the chest.

♦ **settings: Notice of required expert**

- *Flow Rate* : 6-10 l/min for the new-born, 10 to 20 l/min for the infant child.
- *Frequency* of 5-15 Hz (900/min).
- *Peak to peak pressure or ΔP* = in practice 35-50 cmH2O, in case of ARDS ↑ up to maximum 90 cmH2O.
- Direct adjustment of the average pressure.
- *Ti* = 30 to 50%.
- *FR and Δp* are modified as a function of the capnie and FiO2 and P average in function of the oxygenation.

The high-frequency ventilation is often associated with the use of *inhaled nitric oxide (NO)* in the case of pulmonary arterial hypertension (PAH). NO is a specific vasodilator of pulmonary vessels, it has the effect of lowering the pulmonary pressures and Resistors pulmonary vascular.

The needs in No. vary from 5 to 20 ppm. The Administer by connecting the manometer tubing of the bottle of No., the circuit between inspiratory the humidifier and the fitting of the probe of intubation (Coob).

Calculation of the flow of No. in the absence of monitoring device of No. during a transport:

$$\text{débit NO} = \frac{(\text{NO inhalé en ppm}) \times \text{débit du ventilateur}}{(\text{bouteille de NO en ppm})}$$

>>> The transport module with integrated respirator

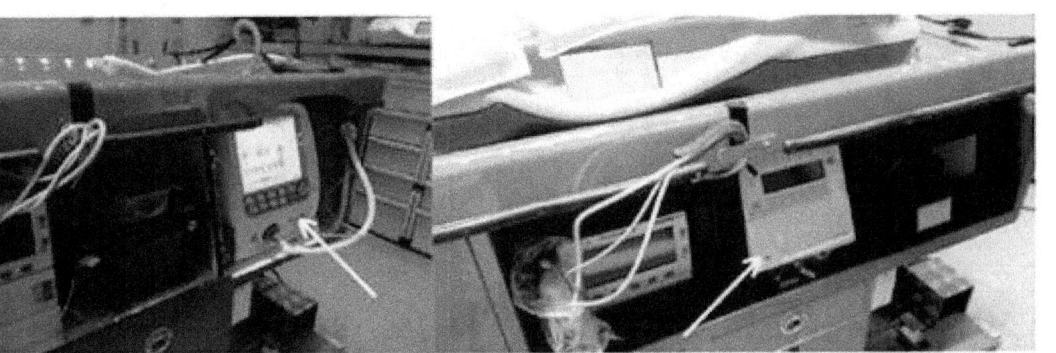

© A.M./N.L.

Think About It

• Adapt the caliber of the ventilatory circuit to the weight of the Child (< 20 kg: pipe of small diameter).

• The use of a heater to heated water allows A humidification and a warming of the gases providing a comfort not negligible and a benefit in the Supported respiratory (limit the broncho-constriction, maintains the airway identified, reduces the risk of respiratory infection).

• The heaters current humidifiers are equipped with thermal probes in the circuits with feedback control of the temperature. The feedback control varies between 33.5 and 42 °C for a humidity to 33 mgH2O/l. They must be adjusted according to the ventilatory mode (NIV, mechanical ventilation). The HFO Request a preset in the factory or the biomedical.

• The respiratory assistance Extra-body (areca nut/ECMO) is a technique that allows you to put the lungs at rest when the state of the pulmonary patient responds neither to the conventional ventilation nor to the high-frequency ventilation. This is an alternative method of short duration.

- In transport, it is practiced the ECMO Veino-arterial (jugulo carotid-) in case of failure or hemodynamic ECMO Veino-venous (jugulo-femoral artery). Among the child less than 6 years of age, the circuits are prepared with blood reconstituted, to the difference of the ECMO of the adult or the boot is done with the physiological serum. The first is vascular surgical. There is very little of mobile units of circulatory support (UMAC) pediatric.

Memo   **58**

Non invasive ventilation

I ♦ Definition
Alternative to mechanical ventilation, the *non invasive ventilation (NIV)* is a method of ventilation in positive pressure. Very widely practiced in neonatology, it is also used in the EMS since several years for infants and older children. It requires of the teams trained Asking well the indications and recognizing the time of passage of a mechanical ventilation.

♦ Indications
- Respiratory distress of the new-born.
- Broncho-alveolitis of the infant.
- Acute Decompensation of chronic respiratory insufficiency.
- Ild of the immunocompromised.
- Thoracic Syndrome acute.
- Acute Asthma serious.
- Drowning.

♦ Contraindications
- Cardiopulmonary arrest.
- Multi-system organ failure.
- Disorders of consciousness (not for the protection of airway), except in the case of apnea in bronchiolitis.
- Facial trauma.
- Obstruction of the upper airway (tumor).
- Pneumothorax not drained.

♦ Benefits
- Avoids additional resistance of the probe of intubation to the accumulation of gas.
- Decreases the work of the respiratory muscles.
- Improves alveolar ventilation.
- Improves the gaseous exchange.

II Technical ♦

A. Equipment

♦ For newborns and infants

The Machines:

• Barometric Respirators carvers of flows adapted to transportation :
- *Mode VS-PEP* : mode of spontaneous ventilation with Positive End Expiratory Pressure (CPAP);
- *Mode bi-phasic* : Mode of ventilation with spontaneous inspiratory assistance and Positive End Expiratory Pressure (BIPAP), called mode "DuoPAP" on some Respirators, with or without respiratory frequency imposed minimum (ST mode).
• *For premature or new-born at term:* Generators of pressures and *generators of pressures to variable flow* (type infant FLOW® driver) with 1 level of pressure (PEP very stable and reliable) or with 2 levels of pressure. These generators can be included or not in respirators. The masks with effects "Coandā" are specific to the infant FLOW®. The heaters humidifiers are indispensable.

The interfaces and circuits:
There are a lot of equipment and different interfaces, adapted to the morphology of the child.
• Nasal cannulas or nasal mask: the choice between these devices is done according to the morphology of the Child, the tolerance of the interface and the effectiveness of the ventilation.
• Harness or bonnet: take the measures head circumference in order to have a bonnet of suitable size, the latter must encompass fully the skull of the Child, to ensure that the ears are not bent.
• Flexible Extension.
• Ventilation Circuit with thermal probes connected to the heater and the generator of pressures or to the respirator of transport.

>>> Model of NIV with nasal cannulas and harness

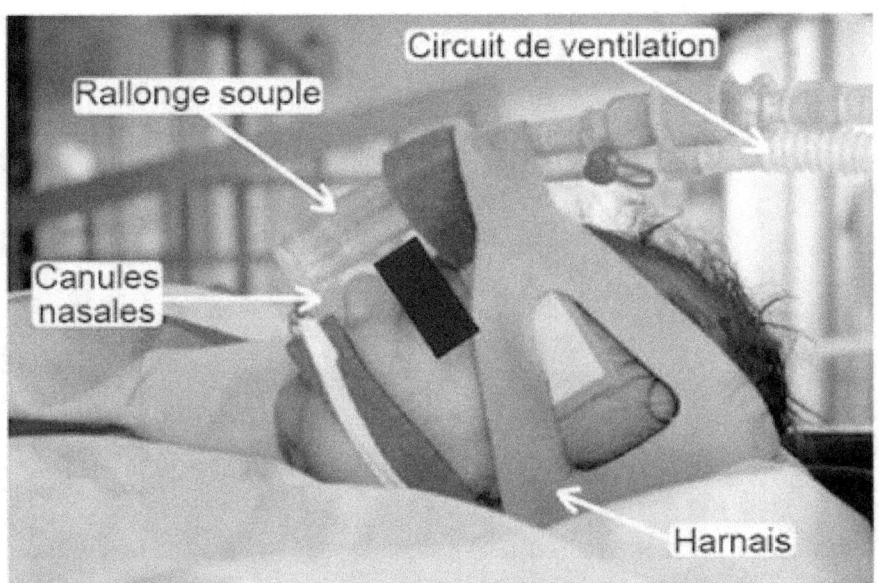

© A.M./N.L.

>>> Model of NIV (Neonatal) with bonnet and nasal mask (left) and NAV with harnesses and nasal mask (right)

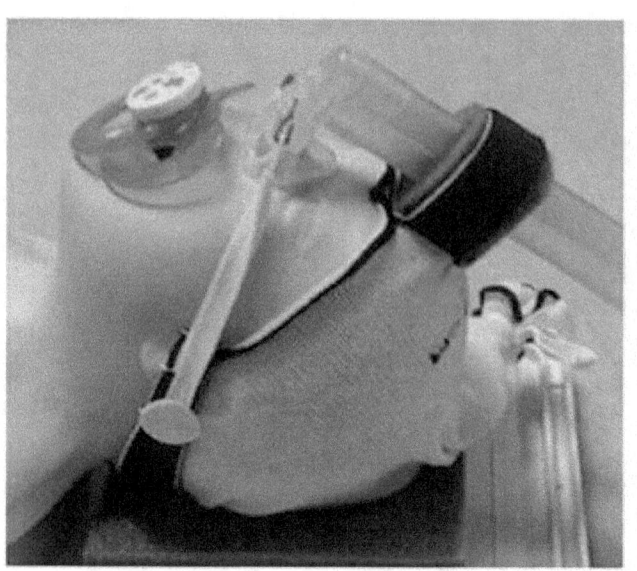 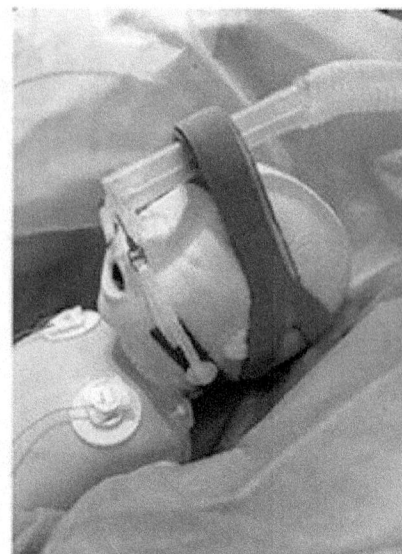

© A.M./N.L.

Other materials:

• Nasal probes uni- or bi-narinaires (Disadvantages: important leakage and poor tolerance of this device).
• The use of the nipple allows you to limit the leaks.
• The use of humidifier heater is recommended for new-born babies and infants.

♦ **For infants > 6-8 kg and children**

The Machines:

• Respirators *to* allow turbine a breakdown invasive and non-invasive of quality, for adults and pediatrics.
• Respirators *tires* including 3rd generation are deprecated (VT and FiO2 unreliable, trigger not suitable).

The modes:

• Mode VS-PEP.

• *Mode bi-phasic* : Mode of ventilation with spontaneous inspiratory assistance and Positive End Expiratory Pressure (BIPAP), with or without respiratory frequency imposed minimum (ST mode).

The interfaces and circuits:
• Nasal Mask or mask oral-nasal (different sizes: XS, S, M, L. There are several brands which sizes are a little different. Find the system which covers the needs).

• Harness.

• Ventilation circuit connected to the respirator of transport: Two types of caliber of pipes are necessary, one for child < 20 kg and the other for child > 20 kg.
• The disadvantage is the absence of heater-humidifier.

>>> VNI model with half mask connected to the ventilation circuit

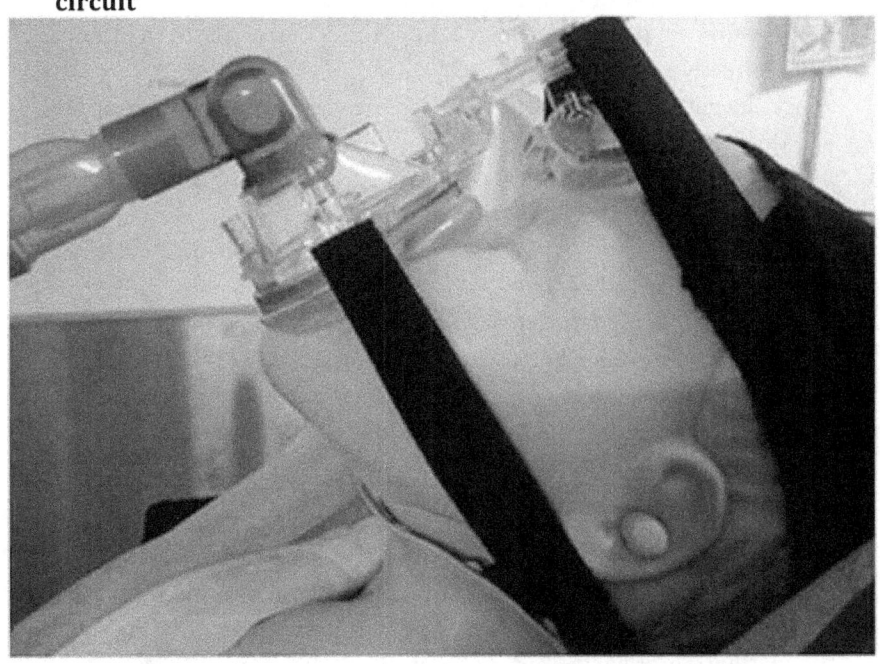

© A.M./N.L.

B. Installation
• Put the child in proclive to 30°.

→ to the newborn/infant :
- According to the degree of urgency, protect the skin with dressings hydrocolloid impressions in order to avoid injuries due to the support of the interface;
- Measure head circumference and position the bonnet or harness adapted to the size of the child;
- Install the mask or the cannula on the flexible extension and adapt the interface (mask/cannula and extension) to the harness/bonnet.

→ *for the child/adolescent* : take the measures of the mask and the position with the help of his harness.

• Connect the device to the ventilatory circuit.
• After s be assured of the proper functioning of the circuit (connection and settings), adapt the device on the child.
• To ensure the proper sealing of the interface in order to maintain a PEP effective.
• Install a gastric probe in the infant to prevent gastric distension.
• In the case of agitation, sedation possible: Midazolam (25 mcg/kg intravenous, intrarectal intranasal or) ±Ketamine (0.2 mg/kg) or Atarax® per os (1 mg/kg/day: period of action 15 min).

→ *For the new-born* : In the case of apnea > 10 seconds, caffeine citrate 20 mg/kg intravenous.

• Monitoring during transport: monitoring, TcPCO2, clinical state of the Child (coloration, signs of a struggle, consciousness). Assess the effectiveness of the NIV, decline in the respiratory rate in the first hour, decline in the TcPCO2, objective SpO2 ≥ 94%, adapt the FiO2.

C. Modes and Settings
→ *for new-born* : PEP + 4, + 5 cmH2O (max = + 6), FiO2 according to the SpO2 required for the term and the age. A specialized opinion is necessary with criteria of FiO2 according to the term and the pathology to decide the intubation, of assisted ventilation and the instillation of surfactant. In some cases the infant FLOW® to 2 levels of pressure is used.

→ *For infants, NCPAP: bronchiolitis +++, obstacle dynamics of airway, ACUTE EDEMA lung, heart failure, acute asthma serious. A PEP + 7 cmH2O has demonstrated its effectiveness in the bronchiolitis.*
→ *for children and infants* : VS-AI-PEP: neuromuscular disease, cystic fibrosis, acute respiratory insufficiency hypoxémiante, some bronchiolitis, acute asthma serious, some décompensations of congenital heart disease.
= *Initial PEP* : 5-7 cmH2O, ↑ 1 by 1
= *Ai* : 4 cmH2O, ↑ gradually from 2 to 2 according to VT + Clinic
= *Pi* = ai + PEP: 10-18 cmH2O, max 20 cmH2O
= *inspiratory trigger* the more sensitive by avoiding the auto-triggering: 0.3 to 0.5 l/min
= *expiratory Trigger* : 40% to 70% according to pathology
= *slope* 0.15 to 0.2 According to tolerance
Etv = Target : 6-8 ml/kg
• *S/T Mode* : frequency depending on the age and Ti according to the frequency
• *S/T Mode + AVAP* (volume guaranteed) for some respirators

D. Other systems to deliver a PEP

♦ **glasses at high flow of fluids such OPTIFLOW®**
Device for glasses to deliver a mix of air-oxygen associated with a PEP. Alternative between the oxygen therapy and the NCPAP often used in Neonatology in withdrawal of the infant FLOW® (mixture air/O2 or air alone to maintain a PEP) or for bronchiolitis little harsh at a flow rate of 2 l/kg/min of a mixture air/O2 (corresponding to 1 PEP ≈ 4 cmH2O) unreliable. Among the larger child a flow to 1 l/kg/min is proposed. There are several devices high speeds, some are with integrated heaters and other not.

♦ *Glasses RAM type cannula®*
Glasses of different sizes for newborns, infants connected to the circuit with heater of respirator carver of flows in mode VS-PEP. This device is used in the weaning mode in the Transfers interhospitaliers output of resuscitation.

Think About It

• **The use of the NIV** in transport induces a fluid consumption very important, thinking to anticipate the transport.

• **The use of a heater** allows A humidification and a warming of the gases providing a comfort not negligible and a benefit in the Supported respiratory (limit the broncho-constriction, maintains the airway identified, reduces the risk of respiratory infections and contributes to the maintenance of the normothermia in the premature).

Memo 59
Track intra-bone

I ♦ Definition
Track of emergency the infant and child, used as a priority when stopping cardio-respiratory (CAB), state of shock or severe dehydration. Among the seriously ill child, in order not to delay the implementation of the treatment, go to the track intra-bone (IO) if failure of track peripheral venous (VVP) after 1 minute (ILCOR 2015) and/or 2 failures of VVP.

♦ Benefits
- *The* vessels the sinusoids of the medullary cavity equivalents of a vein which is not collabe not, even in a state of shock.
- Red Marrow in children less than 6 years.
- Speed of installation.
- The dosage of injected treatments is the same as for the intravenous route.
- The levies are possible: only Ca, K, and PO2 are not correlated with blood rate.

♦ Disadvantages
- Rare complications: diffusion in the tissues, tissue necrosis (more frequent in the case of injection of amines), syndrome of the Lodges++, osteomyelitis and tibial fracture.
- Track intra-bone must be quickly relayed as soon as this is possible by another track first.
- After a failed installation, the IO cannot be reinstalled on the same OS.

♦ Contraindications
- Infection on the site poses, fracture or suspicion on the member.
- Track recent IO ≤ 48 h.
- Prosthetic material.
- Congenital Osteopathy.

II Technical ♦

♦ Hardware

- Compresses.
- Antiseptic.
- Dressing of fixation.
- 10 ml syringe.
- Physiological serum.
- Line of infusion (small fitting, valve 3 track and long tubing).
- Syringe.
- Intraosseous needle (size infant/pediatric/adult).
- Device intra-bone (different models: pistol IO, drill IO...).

♦ insertion sites

1. *Proximal tibia - site to focus in the infant and the child* : at the level of the anterior face-internal The tibia = 1 cm below and inside of the tibial tuberosity earlier or 2 fingers (3 cm) under the base of the ball joint (lunge and external rotation).

2. *Distal tibia* : 1 to 2 cm above the protruding part of the medial malleolus of the tibia.

3. *Proximal femur (< 6 years)* : anterior face of the femur, 1 cm above the ball joint, 1 cm inside of the median line.

4. *Proximal humerus (> 6 years)* : 2 fingers below the OS coracoïde on the humeral tuberosity, arm on the abdomen, elbow adduction, insertion to 45° to the horizontal.

>>> insertion sites

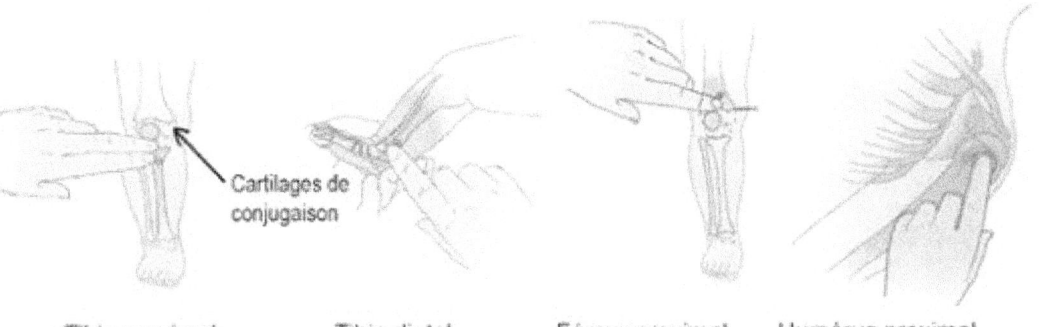

Tibia proximal   Tibia distal   Fémur proximal   Humérus proximal

© Téléflex

♦ **Choice of the size of the needle**
It is done according to the age of the child but the needles of the intra-bone motorised type EZ-IO® are classified in relation to the weight of the child. However, for an optimal placement of the needle IO, it is preferable to refer to the black mark of the needle, and not the weight of the Child : the black mark to 5 mm from the base determines the length of the appropriate needle. If this mark is not visible above the skin (before operate the drill) it must take a needle longer, it decreases the risk of extravasation, incorrect positioning of the needle in the OS.

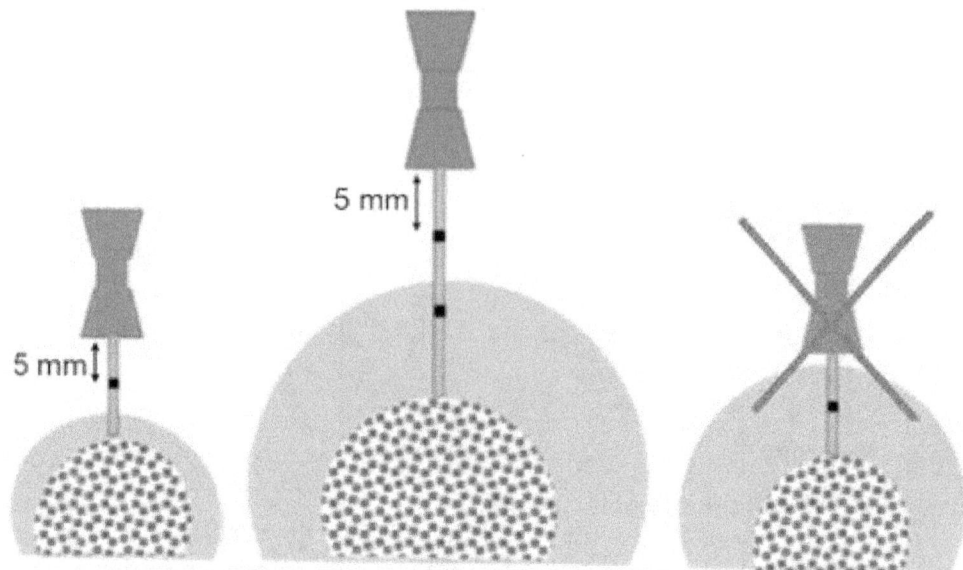

→ *Choice of the size of the COOK®* : 18g < 18 months and 16G > 18 months.

Technical ♦
The technique of poses with the motorized model EZ-IO® allows a better control the operator experienced little thanks to its ease of use.
• Box to needles in close proximity.
• Strict asepsis: cleaning of hands, port of gloves, disinfection of the Insertion Area.
• Purge the infusion line.
• Prepare a syringe of 10 ML OF PHYSIOLOGICAL SALINE connected to the first fitting of the intra-bone: It will serve to test the track and to push in the medullary cavity.
• Good position of the operator and of the Child: for the face antero-internal of the proximal tibia, install the member in bending on a log placed under the knee (or use a pair to maintain the member in position).
• Check that the mandrel dissociates itself well to the needle before inserting the track IO.

• Insert the intra-bone. Push the needle by keeping a vertical angle in relation to the OS. Do not press in the asking, carefully guide the install and stop when there is a release, a decrease of the resistors of the needle.
→ If IO Cook type®, a movement of "Drilling" is necessary to achieve the medullary cavity.
• Once in the medullary cavity, remove the mandrel by unscrewing the upper part and now with the other hand the needle attached in the OS.

>>> **withdrawal of the mandrel**

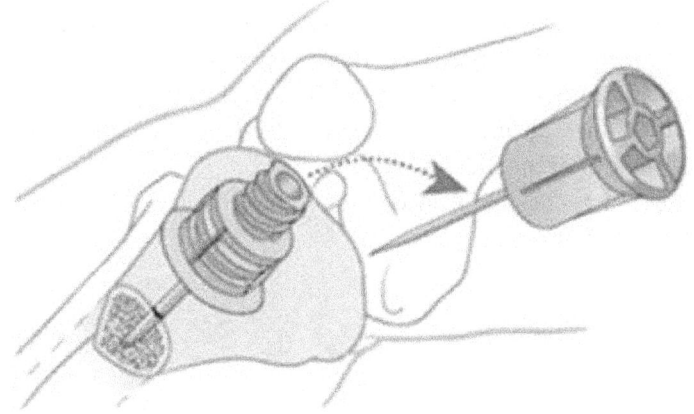

© Téléflex
• Adapt the union bled and test the track using the syringe, 10 ML OF PHYSIOLOGICAL SALINE previously prepared. Try to suck the bone marrow: If the aspiration is possible, slowly inject the 10 ml of physiological saline in order to clean the needle of bone fragment and bone marrow (5 ml in the infant).
• Secure with dressings adapted to the IO to allow for a stabilization of the track. In the case of the use of a dressing adapted to the device EZ-IO® : install the kit without the secure Before tighten the extension of bleeding; if put secondarily: risk of travel.

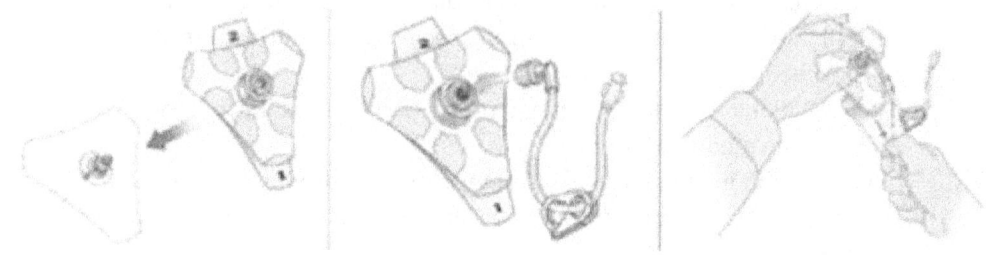

© Téléflex

- If reflux present and flush done without difficulty, then connect the rest of the tubing, it is to be noted that it is preferable to put the infusion rate under pressure (use a syringe pushes for tracks IO, infusion rate for the tibial track: 40 ml/min).
- Monitor the absence of extravasation during the time of establishment of the intra-bone.
- As soon as possible (filling performed, drugs injected...) ask another track first.

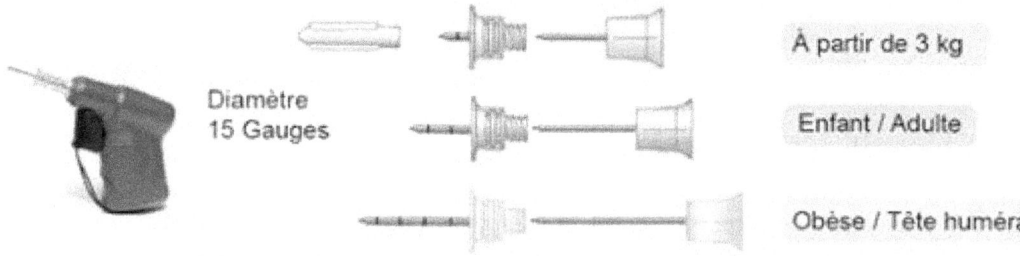

© Téléflex

>>> intra-bone Cook®

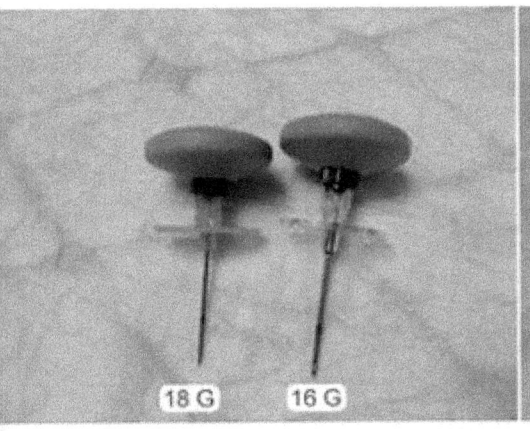 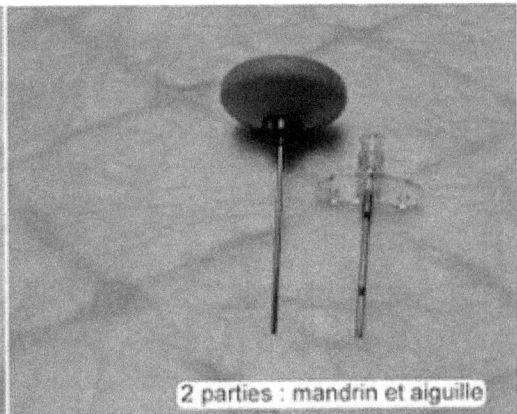

© A.M./N.L.

Think About It

• The needle is well asked if:

- Immobile in the OS (in vertical position);

- Aspiration of blood or bone marrow to the syringe;

- Absence of extravasation after injection of 5 to 10 ml of physiological saline to slow flow;

- Absence of resistors of infusion.

• Caution: The medullary space is narrow at the small infant.

• Increased surveillance of the anterior and posterior (risk of transfixion of the Os).

• If the child is conscious and reactive, anesthetize locally (Xylocaine® 1%).

• The IO does not pass to the IRM.

♦ **withdrawal of the device**

>>> withdrawal of the device

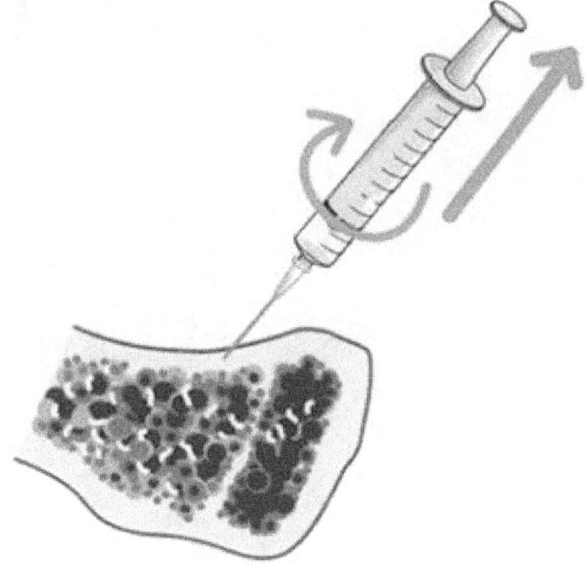

- Take a syringe 10 ml or 20 ml (Luer Lock®) and screw on the needle.
- Turn in a clockwise direction by pulling.
- Simple dressing.

Memo

Umbilical track

I ♦ Definition
The installation of *catheter umbilical venous (KTVO)* is a medical act, made during resuscitation or vital distress in the newborn and if failure of the installation of venous track device. It is a track easily accessible, it is contemplated up to the eighth day of life.

II Technical ♦

♦ Preparation of equipment
• Tangled Field (prepared around the navel).
• Sterile FIELD NOT holes (to install the hardware).

• Scalpel.
• Umbilical Arterial Catheter (n° 3.5 < 1 000 g and No. 5 > 1 000 g).
• Cock 3 tracks.
• Wires to skin, needle curve.
• Dressings STÉRI type-strip®.
• Sterile gloves.
• Sponges and skin antiseptic.
• Sterile instruments: scissors, clip and needle holder.
• Syringe of 5 ml pre-filled with the physiological serum.
• Prepare a line of infusion (small fitting, valve 3 track and long tubing).

Technical ♦
• Installation of the Child, maintain the hands and legs of the newborn during the care.
• Washing of hands, port of sterile gloves.
• Asepsis of the skin: according to the Protocol of the service (antiseptic BISEPTINE type® more widespread in Pediatrics).
• Position the tangled field.
• Adapt the umbilical arterial catheter to the 3-way lever valve and bleed the assembly with the physiological serum.

- Position around the umbilicus a loose ligation ready to be tightened in the case of bleeding abundant (use a gastric probe or a probe of aspiration of small caliber).
- Cut the cord to 1.5-2 cm of the skin using a scalpel.
- Using the pliers sterile, perform a slight pull on the cord and locate the umbilical vessels (1 vein and 2 arteries).
- Insert the catheter previously served in the umbilical vein, up to observe a reflux of blood to the aspiration, then rinse with the syringe of 5 ml of physiological saline (ensure that there is no leak from the umbilical vein).

→ *central position* : (1.5 × weight (kg)) + 5.5) radio control required to verify the location of the catheter.

→ *position device* : In case of emergency or if radio impossible, 5 cm for the new-born at term and 3 cm for the premature.

- *Attach the catheter: Pass the wire in the jelly of Wharton, perform a scholarship around the umbilicus and weaving the Son in "Spartan" around the catheter, make a node and cut the rest of the wire with the chisel sterile. Then secure the "Spartan" with a dressing of type steristrips® placed in "flag" on the node.*
- Then adapt the tubing to the cock 3 tracks (the latter can be used in the event of a blood sample if the catheter is positioned in Central) and start the infusion.

Note: A KTVO asked in emergency will be removed to the arrival in resuscitation to install another in the best conditions

>>> KTVO Journey

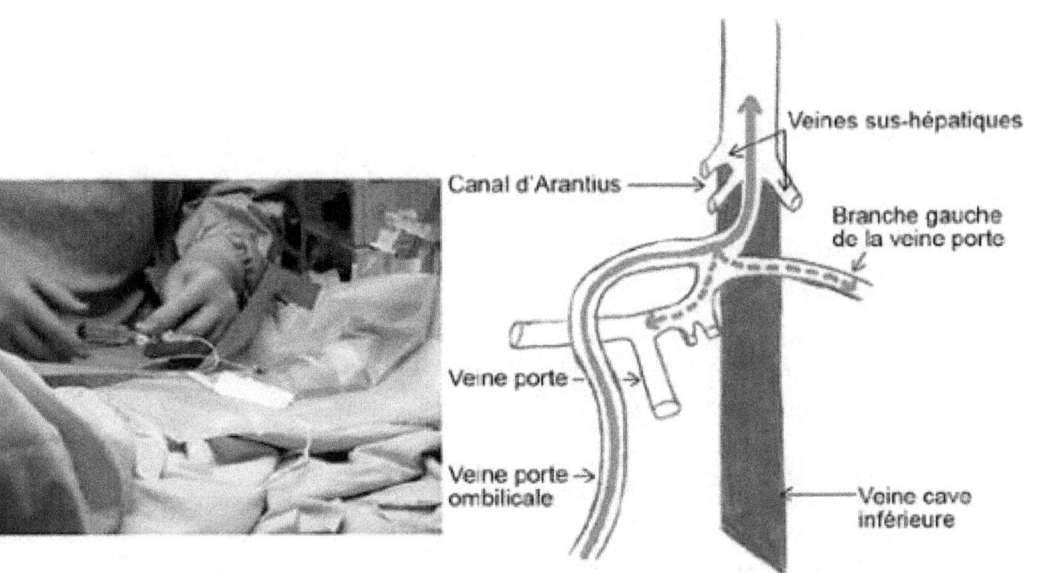

Think About It

• **Monitor the bleeding of the bead after installation** : it is possible to keep the ligature around the umbilicus, in the loosening in small (haemorrhagic risk in the hours which follow the install).

• In the premature, limit the contact time of the antiseptic with the skin because **significant risk of burns.**

• Prior to inject, always **check if there is a reflux.**

Memo 61

Venous track in external jugular

I ♦ Definition
Venous track of emergency when tracks devices are not accessible.

♦ Advantage
Superficial vein of large caliber, often the most easy to identify and to cathétériser in case of hypovolemia.

♦ Disadvantages
• The position when installing a track in external jugular is not always well tolerated.
• Difficulty of access when cardio-pulmonary resuscitation.
• The anatomy of the neck of the infant makes its catheterization difficult.
• *Flow rate of infusion in positional function of the position of the head.*

II Technical ♦

♦ Hardware
• Box to needles.

• Compresses.

• Antiseptic.

• Dressings of type steri-strip®, TEGADERM®.
• Syringe of 2 ml of physiological saline to purge the catheter.
• Prepare an upstream line of infusion (small fitting, valve 3 track and long tubing).
• Catheters.

Technical ♦
• Auscultate and check the bilateral character of the vesicular murmur.
• Maintain the Child on the back, the head in the extension of 30° (use a Billot if needed).

- Position the head of the child toward the left hand side, use the external jugular vein right of preference.
- Washing of hands and port of gloves.
- Disinfect the puncture site on, anesthetize locally according to the degree of urgency.
- Use a catheter short for a first device.
- Compress The external jugular vein above the clavicle for it to become more visible.
- Bite in now a angle of 10°, up to feel a release when the needle between in the light of the vein.
- Connect the tubing.
- Secure with a dressing of type TEGADERM®.

Think About It

Disadvantage: is only visible when the external jugular vein crosses by in before the muscle sternocléidomastoïdien.

Memo 62

Track peripheral venous

I ♦ Definition
The installation of a venous track device is to introduce a catheter in a vein. The morphology of the Child, hypovolemia, the States of shock, the vessels of low diameters can make it difficult for them to put in place.

II Technical ♦

♦ Preparation upstream
• Put in trust.
• Inform the care.
• If the conditions permit: Use the distraction, (Mark the centers of the interests of the child), use the means painkillers: nitrous oxide, sucrose for infants, cream anesthésiante (duration of installation of 1 h, difficult to use in préhospitalier).
• Leave a place to parents, if possible.
• Organize before the CARE (hardware and role of each).

♦ procedure
• Good installation of the Child and the caregiver.
• Preparation of equipment:
- Box to needles ;
- Compresses;
- Antiseptic;
- Withers of appropriate size;
- Dressings of fixing of type steri-strip®, TEGADERM® ;
- Syringe of 2 ml of physiological saline ;
- Prepare a line of infusion (small fitting, valve 3 track and long tubing);
- Catheters:

Norme	Taille en mm	Débit max	Couleur
24 G	14 mm pour le prématuré 19 mm pour le nouveau-né à terme	13/18 ml/h	Jaune
22 G	25 mm	25/40 ml/h	Bleu
20 G	30 mm	55/65 ml/h	Rose
18 G	32 mm	80/100 ml/h	Vert
16 G	45 mm	160/200 ml/h	Gris
14 G	50 mm	270 ml/h	Orange

- Washing of hands, port of gloves.
- Asepsis of the skin: according to the Protocol of the service (antiseptic BISEPTINE type® more widespread in Pediatrics).

Neonatology	Pediatrics
• BISPETINE® 1re application; • Drying by buffering with compresses sterile ; • BISPETINE® 2e application; • Respect of contact time of 30 seconds; • Rinse with sterile water; • Drying by buffering with compresses sterile ;	• BISPETINE® 1re application; • Drying by buffering with compresses sterile ; • BISPETINE® 2e application; • Spontaneous drying;

- Main venous approaches:

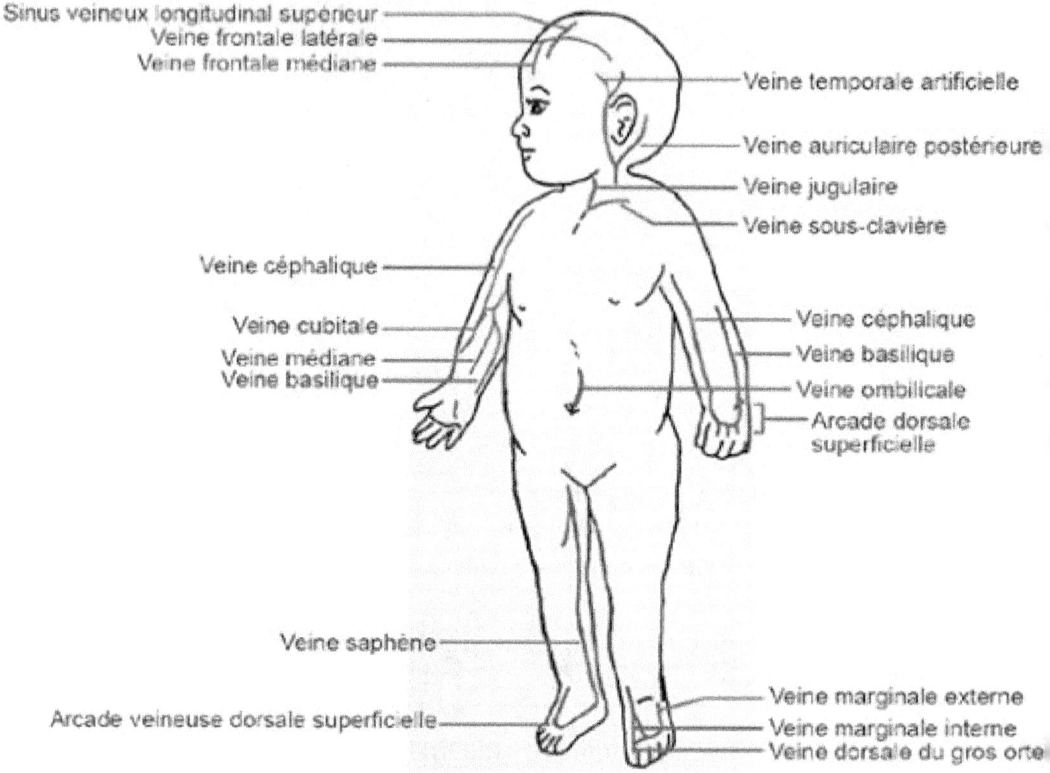

Sinus veineux longitudinal supérieur
Veine frontale latérale
Veine frontale médiane

Veine temporale artificielle
Veine auriculaire postérieure
Veine jugulaire
Veine sous-clavière

Veine céphalique

Veine cubitale
Veine médiane
Veine basilique

Veine céphalique
Veine basilique
Veine ombilicale
Arcade dorsale superficielle

Veine saphène

Arcade veineuse dorsale superficielle

Veine marginale externe
Veine marginale interne
Veine dorsale du gros orte

→ In infants, the outskirts such venous that the superficial veins are more difficult to achieve because of adipose tissue more important that hides the veins.

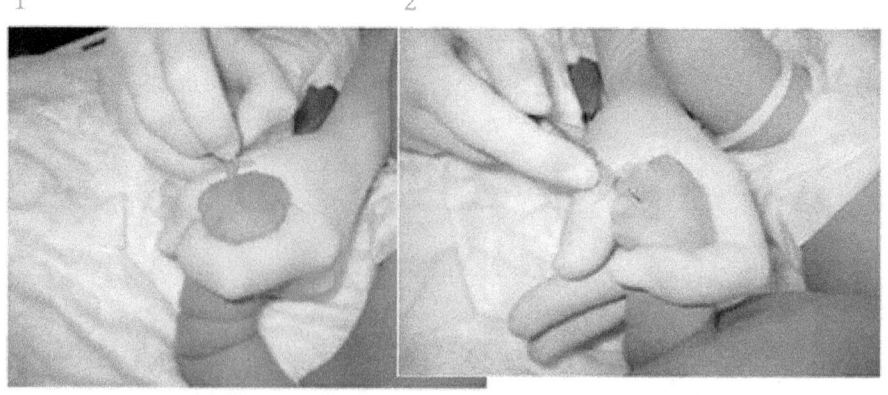

- Good installation (adequate lighting, good maintenance: the newborn, put the wrist in bending between the thumb and the index = withers natural).
- Identify the vein and prick.
- Fit the catheter as soon as in reflux of blood is visible: either with the needle guide, either without the needle to the syringe of 2 ml pre-filled of physiological serum which serves as the liquid mandrel (This method allows a manipulation more soft for the fragile veins, smaller sizes, as in neonates).
- (Re)Test the permeability of the track with the syringe of 2 ML OF PHYSIOLOGICAL SALINE once the catheter mounted.

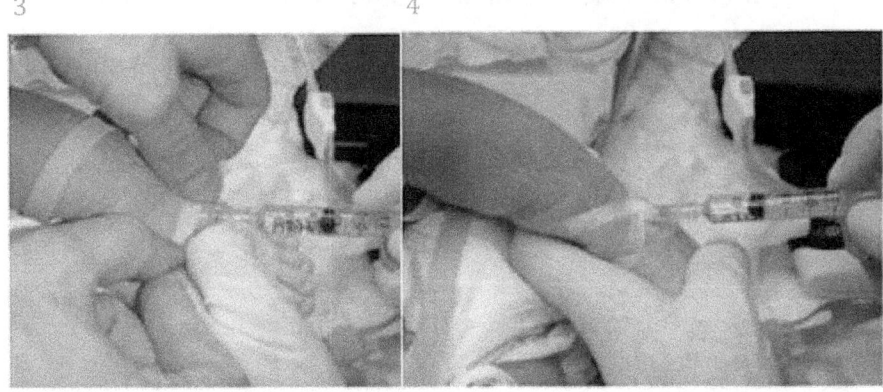

3 4

- Fixation with dressings of type
- Fixation in tie.

steri-strip®

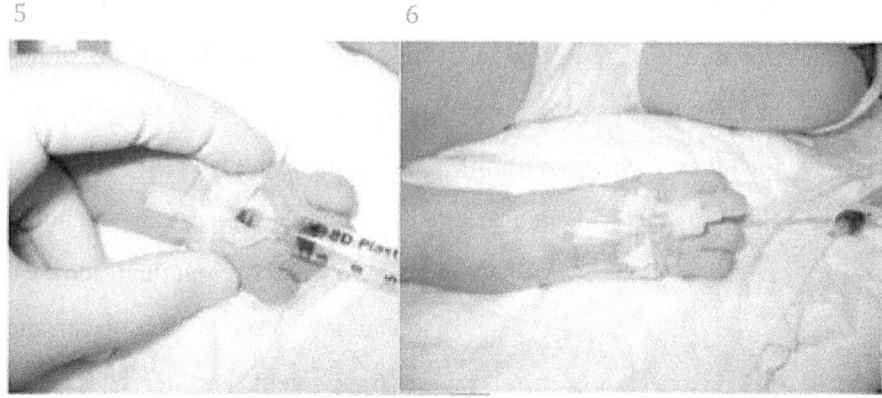

5 6

- Test for leaks again after the mounting.
- Position the dressing of type TEGADERM® in a non-circular.

Think about it:

Attention +++: not of free flow in the Child (always use a syringe).

- No levy, of taking the voltage or saturation positioned in the perfused member.
- Always monitor the puncture site: induration, seepage, redness, flow.
- In case of failure of installing or cardiopulmonary arrest, to quickly put a track intra-bone (see Mémo 59) except in neonatology: Install a umbilical arterial catheter (see Mémo 60).

Part 3

The hygiene rules

>>> Mémo 63 - Asepsie

>>> Mémo 64 - Hygiène

>>> Mémo 65 - Nettoyage et désinfection de l'ambulance

Memo 63

Asepsis.

I ♦ Definition
The asepsis. affects all of the hygiene measures and precautions build in place before, during and after an act invasive (install catheter, track peripheral venous, dressing).
In préhospitalier, it will adapt to the places of the intervention, while respecting the maximum hygiene rules.

II ♦ the hygiene of hands
• **SHA in préhospitalier:** Not having point of water, the friction of hands by hydro-alcoholic solution will be the most common technique used before and after each act.
• **The Port of Gloves:** for each act in contact with biological fluids. Sterile gloves in préhospitalier will be them used for the acts to achieve in sterile (install arterial catheter or central, urinary probe).
• **The washing of hands:** it will be carried out with a mild soap as soon as possible. Before the beginning of the intervention, on arrival at the hospital and in return for intervention.

III ♦ antiseptics

They aim to eliminate the transient flora and resistant present on the skin. The steps and their uses are different depending on the desired objective.

Level of the infectious risk	Objectives	Technique of détersion
Important (installing a VVC)	Eliminate the transient flora Reduce the resistant Flora	In 4 time with 2 badigeons
Medium (installing a VVP long-term)	Eliminate the transient flora	In 4 time with 1 whitewash or an antiseptic 2 time
Low (installing a VVP in the short term)	Reduce the transient flora	An antiseptic 1 time (on visually skin own). In pediatrics, antiseptic 2 time.

• **Steps 4 Time:** antiseptic iodized type chlorinated or:
- Mechanical détersion;
- Flushing physiological serum ;
- Drying;
- Disinfection (whitewash).

• **Steps 1 or 2 Time:** antiseptic alcoholic type or aqueous-based.

IV ♦ Preparation of the site

According to the act performed, it will use the same precautions that in inpatient, such as:
- The shearing of the site if necessary;
- A wide disinfection procedures;

- A sterile field;
- A bandage or sterile film.

Think About It

The holding of the smuriste is to change as many times as necessary during its care (patient BMR or at risk, defiled by biological fluids, earth, oil...).

Memo 64

Hygiene

I ♦ Definition
Hygiene practices in préhospitalier are the same in adults and the child: washing of hands, port of gloves, cleaning of the equipment between the transport. However, the pediatrics, and more particularly the neonatology, require a few special precautions.

Decree No. 2004-802 of 29 July 2004

Chapter II RULES OF PROFESSIONAL - Section I - Article R. 4312-11

The nurse or the nurse respects and enforces the rules of hygiene in the administration of care, in the use of material and in the holding of the premises. It ensures the proper disposal of solid and liquid waste resulting from its acts professionals.

II Technical ♦

♦ **aseptic technique during transport**
• Bare Hands: Not of Jewel, not varnished, nails short.
• Washing of hands: hydro-alcoholic solution (only on hands not soiled, not wet, do not rinse, nor wipe).

- Port of gloves and mask during of the invasive care: track laying peripheral venous, contact with bodily secretions (suction, installing gastric probe, pocket to urine).
- In neonatology, wear a surblouse non sterile single-use. In a room of the birth, add the Charlotte, the mask and shoe covers.
- Stringent precautions when handling the sterile equipment (sterile gloves, mask, blouse).
- Put a mask when the child is infected (or suspicion of lung infection): Insulation air/contact/droplets. In addition, during primary intervention (intervention in the home or in public places), the pathology of the child is not always known.
- Washing of hands after each care and at the end of each supported.
- Disposal of waste in the chain adapted.

between Transport
- Make a friction hydro-alcoholic of hands.
- Port of gloves and a surblouse.
- Clean with a disinfectant detergent non-toxic validated by the direction of the institution:
- The incubator or the mattress shell;
- The surfaces, the wrists and the facades of the module or of the stretcher;
- The rickshaw-syringes;
- The equipment used (respirator, scope, cables and connectors in contact with the patient, etc.).
- Leave to dry, remove the personal protective equipment (gloves, surblouse) and repeat a friction hydro-alcoholic of hands.
- Make the traceability of the equipment.

daily and weekly cleaning operations
Complete cleaning of the mobile unit (hospital UMH) with a disinfectant detergent non-toxic validated by the direction of the institution:
- Inside and Outside, cab front and rear (clean surfaces, wrists, armchairs and facades);
- The weekly disinfection concerns the aspiration of the inside of the cab, the cleaning of the walls, surfaces, the inside of the

cupboards and drawers as well as the maintenance of the refrigerator.

◆ exceptional cleaning
- For the insulation (waste and cleaning), specific fact sheets to each structure are developed: refer to them to know the appropriate personal protective equipment and precautions to take (insulation BMR, protective insulation, etc.).
- Specific Decontamination: for example the VRS, highly contagious virus in pediatrics, responsible for many bronchiolitis (mode of transmission by droplets/contact): resists 30 minutes on the skin and 6-7 hours on the linen and objects.

Think About It

- When all disinfections begin by the more own toward the more dirty.

- Do not use iodized antiseptic in the newborn and the infant of less than 1 months. In addition, it is not recommended to use for a prolonged period of time in the home of the Child on the mucous membranes or the large surfaces (risk of allergy, passage of the iodine in the blood).

- In the case of BMR, VRS... change the expiratory block of the respirator.

Memo   **65**

Cleaning and disinfection of the Ambulance

I ◆ daily maintenance of the driving position
- **Seats and soil:** aspire methodically (body of the vacuum cleaner to the outside of the vehicle).
- **Table Panel, gear lever, handbrake, interior doors and handles, radio, micro, seats:** Clean with a detergent-disinfectant

for floors, surfaces and movable property and an absorbent support single-use.
• **Soil:** wash the soil with a detergent-disinfectant for floors, surfaces and movable property.

II ♦ Maintenance of the cell health after each use
• **Sharps:** in a specific manifold closed on a provisional basis.

Single use materials, waste of activities of care, household waste: evacuate in bags closed according to the sector adequate.

• **Vacuum mattress, stretcher, foot to serum, seats of attendants:** Clean with a detergent-disinfectant for floors, surfaces and movable property, as well as a absorbent support single-use.
• **Mobile Device of oxygen, suction device of the mucosities:** Clean with a detergent-disinfectant for floors, surfaces and movable property compatible with the material and an absorbent support single-use.
• **Medical Device: reusable** clean-disinfect it with a detergent-disinfectant without rinsing for medical device, compatible with the material, and a absorbent support single-use. Evacuate in a sealed packaging pending the cleaning/disinfection by dipping at the base.
• **Door handles:** Clean with a detergent-disinfectant for floors, surfaces and movable property and an absorbent support single-use.

III ♦ maintenance daily and weekly for the health cell
• **Vertical walls:** Clean with a detergent-disinfectant for floors, surfaces and movable property, as well as a absorbent support single-use.
• **Windows:** clean with the product for Windows. Use a detergent-disinfectant for floors, surfaces and movable property in the case of biological soiling.
• **Soil:** Remove any dust from the ground. Aspire to in leaving the body of the vacuum cleaner to the outside of the vehicle to the extent possible or perform a scan wet. Wash the soil with a detergent-disinfectant for floors, surfaces and movable property.

- **Collectors of sharps:** close the manifold (final closure), evacuate, according to the circuit of waste arising from care activities involving infectious risks.
- **Drawers and cupboards:** any empty. Clean with a detergent-disinfectant for floors, surfaces and movable property, as well as a absorbent support single-use.
- **Equipment of the cell health** : any exit. Clean-disinfect it with a detergent-disinfectant for medical device.
- The **mouths of blowing and air extraction:** aspire. Clean with a detergent-disinfectant for floors, surfaces and movable property, as well as a absorbent support single-use.
- Multiresistant bacteria (BMR): see *Mémo 64 Hygiène*.

Part 4

Pharmacology

>>> Mémo 66 - Acétate de désoxycortone

>>> Mémo 67 - Aciclovir

>>> Mémo 68 - Acide tranexamique

>>> Mémo 69 - Adénosine

>>> Mémo 70 - Adénosine triphosphate

>>> Mémo 71 - Adrénaline (épinéphrine)

>>> Mémo 72 - Alprostadil

>>> Mémo 73 - Amikacine

>>> Mémo 74 - Amiodarone

>>> Mémo 75 - Amoxicilline

>>> Mémo 76 - Atracurium

>>> Mémo 77 - Atropine

>>> Mémo 78 - Bétaméthasone

>>> Mémo 79 - Bircabonate de sodium

>>> Mémo 80 - Bromure de rocuronium

>>> Mémo 81 - Bromure de vérocuronium

>>> Mémo 82 - Bromure d'ipratropium

>>> Mémo 83 - Céfotaxime

>>> Mémo 84 - Ceftriaxone

>>> Mémo 85 - Charbon activé

>>> Mémo 86 - Clonazépam

>>> Mémo 87 - Crème anesthésiante

>>> Mémo 88 - Diazépam

>>> Mémo 89 - Dobutamine

>>> Mémo 90 - Dopamine

>>> Mémo 91 - Ésoméprazole

>>> Mémo 92 - Étomidate

>>> Mémo 93 - Fentanyl

>>> Mémo 94 - Flumazénil

>>> Mémo 95 - Fosphénytoïne

>>> Mémo 96 - Furosémide

>>> Mémo 97 - Gentamicine

>>> Mémo 98 - Glucagon

>>> Mémo 99 - Hémisuccinate d'hydrocortisone

>>> Mémo 100 - Hydroxocobalamine

>>> Mémo 101 - Hydroxyzine

>>> Mémo 102 - Ibuprofène

>>> Mémo 103 - Insuline

>>> Mémo 104 - Kétamine

>>> Mémo 105 - Mannitol 10 %

>>> Mémo 106 - Méthylprednisolone

>>> Mémo 107 - Métronidazole

>>> Mémo 108 - Midazolam

>>> Mémo 109 - Morphine

>>> Mémo 110 - N-Acétyl Cystéine

>>> Mémo 111 - Nalbuphine

>>> Mémo 112 - Naloxone

>>> Mémo 113 - Néfopam

>>> Mémo 114 - Nicardipine

>>> Mémo 115 - Noradrénaline

>>> Mémo 116 - Ondansétron

>>> Mémo 117 - Paracétamol

>>> Mémo 118 - Phénobarbital

>>> Mémo 119 - Phénytoïne

>>> Mémo 120 - Propofol

>>> Mémo 121 - Propranolol

>>> Mémo 122 - Protoxyde d'azote

>>> Mémo 123 - Salbutamol

>>> Mémo 124 - Sérum salé hypertonique NaCl 7,5 %

>>> Mémo 125 - Solution sucrée à visée antalgique

>>> Mémo 126 - Sufentanil

>>> Mémo 127 - Sulfate de magnésium

>>> Mémo 128 - Sulfate de morphine

>>> Mémo 129 - Suxaméthonium

>>> Mémo 130 - Terbutaline

>>> Mémo 131 - Thiopental

>>> Mémo 132 - Tramadol

>>> Mémo 133 - Vancomycine

>>> Mémo 134 - Vitamine K1

Memo 66

Acetate of deoxycorticosterone acetate

DCI and name	Acetate of deoxycorticosterone acetate (SYNCORTYL®)
Pharmacological Class	Mineralocorticoid
Indications	Insufficient acute adrenal
Contra-indications	High blood pressure
Side effects	• Hydrosodée retention • High blood pressure • Anaphylactic Shock • Urticaria

Posology	IM: 5 to 10 mg/m2/i To renew according the evolution
Method of administration	Intramuscular (IM)

Memo 67
Aciclovir

DCI and name	**Acyclovir (Zovirax®)**
Pharmacological Class	Antivirals
Indications	Treatment of herpes infections
Contra-indications	• History of hypersensitivity to the aciclovir • Lactose intolerance
Side effects	Rash benign
Posology	IV: 20 mg/kg or 500 mg/m2/8 H
Method of administration	Intravenous (IV)

Memo 68
Tranexamic acid

DCI and name	**Tranexamic acid (EXACYL®)**
Pharmacological Class	Antifibrinolytic
Indications	Massive hemorrhage
Contra-indications	• History of thromboembolic events • Severe renal impairment
Side effects	• Affection of the skin and the skin tissue • Digestive Disorders • Hypotension
Posology	IV: 10-15 mg/kg (max. 1 g) in 10 min, and then 15 mg/kg/8 h
Method of administration	Intravenous (IV)

Adenosine

DCI and name	**Adenosine (KRENOSIN®)**
Pharmacological Class	Endogenous nucleoside with effect peripheral vasodilator antiarrhythmic,

Indications	• Supraventricular tachycardia
Contra-indications	• Atrioventricular block • Long QT Syndrome • Arterial Hypotension Severe **Prefer the STRIADYNE® (if available) in the KRENOSIN®**
Side effects	• Bradycardia • Headache • Dizziness • Anxiety • Anguish • Nausea • Facial Flush • Bronchospasm
Posology	IV: 0.1 mg/kg (max. 6 mg), then 0.2 mg/kg (max. 12 mg)
Method of administration	• Intravenous (IV) • Inject in flush, on venous track device to the upper member left, under control continuous ECG • Keep the atropine ready to provision

Memo 70

Adenosine triphosphate

DCI and name	Adenosine triphosphate (STRIADYNE®)
Pharmacological Class	Endogenous nucleoside with effect peripheral vasodilator antiarrhythmic,
Indications	Junctional tachycardia
Contra-indications	• Atrioventricular block • Malfunction sino-atrial • Asthma
Side effects	• Headache • Dizziness • Anxiety • Nausea • Facial Flush • Bradycardia • Asystole • Dyspnea • Feeling of oppression

Posology	IV: 1 mg/kg (max. 20 mg)
	Inject in flush, on venous track device to the upper member left, under control ECG
	Keep the atropine ready to provision
Method of administration	Intravenous (IV)

Memo 71
Adrenaline (epinephrine)

	Adrenaline (epinephrine)
Pharmacological Class	Adrenergic and dopaminergic,
Indications	• Treatment of cardiac arrest and of the failure and myocardial
	• Treatment of anaphylactic shock, laryngitis,
Contra-indications	• Coronary heart disease
	• Disorders of the rhythm
	• Obstructive cardiomyopathy
Side effects	• Sinus tachycardia
	• Disorders of the rhythm

	• Rarely in the Child: anginal attacks, myocardial infarction
Posology	• IV: 0.01 mg/kg to 0.03 mg/kg as a bolus in the event of a resuscitation of the new-born, or 10 to 30 mcg/kg. • 0.1 mcg/kg/min, continuous infusion and then titration • In the case of ACR in the Child: 0.01 mg/kg • IM (anaphylaxis): 0.01 mg/kg • Nebulization (adrenaline without sulphite): 5 mg Attention: inactivation by bicarbonate
Method of administration	• Intravenous (IV) • Intra-bone (IO) • Intramuscular (IM) • Nebulization (aerosol)

Alprostadil

DCI and name	Alprostadil (Prostin VR®)

Pharmacological Class	Family of prostaglandins E1, fatty acids natural
Indications	Temporary maintenance of the permeability of the ductus arteriosus
Contra-indications	No
Side effects	• Flush • Bradycardia • Fever • Apnea • Diffuse pain
Posology	IV: 0.01-0.05 mcg/kg/min
Method of administration	Intravenous (IV)

Memo

Amikacin

DCI and name	**Amikacin (AMIKLIN®)**
Pharmacological Class	Antibacterial antibiotics of the family of the aminoglycosides
Indications	• Pyélonéphrites and urinary tract infections of febrile infants and young

	children • In association with the cefotaxime if < 3 months
Contra-indications	• Allergy to aminoglycoside antibiotics • In the case of myasthenia gravis • In association with the polymyxins by the parenteral route
Side effects	• Nephrotoxicité (dosage too high, duration of treatment, renal impairment earlier) • Ototoxicity • Allergic Reaction
Posology	• IV new-born: - 30 to 33 Its → 32.5 mg/kg/48 h* - 34 to 36 Its → 30 mg/kg/36 h* - > 37 Its → 27.5 mg/kg/24 to 36 h* * With blood metering • IV child: - Monotherapy: 30 mg/kg/24 h on 30 min - In dual therapy: 15 mg/kg/24 h
Method of administration	Intravenous (IV)

Memo 74
Amiodarone

DCI and name	Amiodarone (CORDARONE®)
Pharmacological Class	Antiarrhythmic Drug, class III
Indications	• Track IV only in case of RTAS with chocable pace after failure of 3e shock and after the injection of adrenaline. • Per OS for the supraventricular tachycardia poorly tolerated and not reduced by the STRIADYNE®
Contra-indications	Attention: the therapeutic dose is near the lethal dose, that is why the Form IV is only used in the cab on Rhythm Disorder
Side effects	Moderate bradycardia
Posology	• PO: - Loading dose: 500 mg/m2/i - Maintenance dose: 75 to 250 mg/m2/i • In the case of ACR with rhythm chocable: 5 mg/kg

Method of administration	• Per os (PO) • Intravenous (IV) only in RTAS with rhythm chocable

Amoxicillin

DCI and name	Amoxicillin (CLAMOXYL®)
Pharmacological Class	Broad-spectrum penicillins
Indications	• Treatment of pneumonitis • Ent Infections • Urinary Tract Infections • Endocardites • Sepsis • Maternal infections fetal-
Contra-indications	• In case of allergy to antibiotics of the family of beta-lactam antibiotics • In the case of phenylketonuria
Side effects	• Diarrhea • Nausea • Rash • Cutanéo Candidiasis anaphylactic-
Posology	IV: - < I7: 50 mg/kg/12 h IVD, infection maternal-fetal with meningeal reached:

	100 mg/kg dose - > J7: 50 mg/kg/8 h IVD
Method of administration	Intravenous (IV)

Memo

Atracurium

DCI and name	Atracurium (TRACRIUM®)
Pharmacological Class	Peripherally acting muscle relaxant
Indications	• Curare depolarizing non • Induction and maintenance of a myorelaxation during anesthesia
Contra-indications	Hypersensitivity to the atracrium or one of its components
Side effects	• Hypotension • Redness of the skin
Posology	IV: induction = 0.6 mg/kg < 2 years: 0.4 mg/kg Continuous = 0.3 to 0.6 mg/kg/h Time limit for action: 1.5-3 Min Duration of action: 45-60 min
Method of administration	Intravenous (IV)

Memo 77

Atropine

DCI	Atropine
Pharmacological Class	Alkaloids of the belladonna: tertiary amines
Indications	Protection of vagal events/bradycardia during induction, anticholinergic antidote
Contra-indications	Hypersensitivity to any of the components
Side effects	Tachycardia
Posology	IV: 20 mcg/kg
Method of administration	Intravenous (IV)

Memo

Betamethasone

DCI and name	Betamethasone (CELÉSTÈNE®)
Pharmacological Class	Glucocorticoid
Indications	• Asthma
	• Laryngitis sub-glottal
Contra-indications	Some viral diseases in Evolution (hepatitis, herpes, chicken pox, herpes zoster)
Side effects	• Euphoria
	• Excitement
	• Rare cases of anaphylaxis
Posology	PO: 20 drops/kg, or 0.25 mg/kg/dose
Method of administration	Per os (PO)

Memo

Bircabonate Of sodium

DCI	Sodium Bicarbonate 14 ‰, 42 ‰
Pharmacological Class	• Product of alkaline contribution • Physiological compound of the plasma
Indications	• Correction of metabolic acidosis documented • Threatening hyperkalemia • Cab
Contra-indications	• Metabolic alkalosis • Respiratory acidosis
Side effects	• Metabolic alkalosis • Hypokalemia in case of overdose
Posology	• IV: 1 mEq/kg Rinse+++ at the abatement • In the new-born, use bicarbonate semi-molar to 42 ‰ (1 mmol = 2 ml) on 5 to 15 min
Method of administration	Intravenous (IV)

Memo

Of bromide rocuronium

DCI and name	Of bromide rocuronium (ESMERON®)
Pharmacological Class	Myorelaxant
Indications	• Curare depolarizing not used in induction during the Tracheal intubation • Used if contraindication to suxamethonium (CÉLOCURINE®)
Contra-indications	• Myasthenia gravis (against-formal indication) • Known hypersensitivity to the active substance or to any of the components
Side effects	• Neuromuscular block extended, anaphylaxis Do not use if absence of Antidote • : Antagonist Sugammadex BRIDION (® : 16 mg/kg)
Posology	IV: 1.2 mg/kg

	Time limit for action: 60 s
	Duration of action: 45 min
Method of administration	• Intravenous (IV)

Memo 81

Of bromide vérocuronium

DCI and name	Of bromide vérocuronium (NORCURON®)
Pharmacological Class	A myorelaxant curare depolarizing non
Indications	Curare indicated in the general anesthesia
Contra-indications	Hypersensitivity to the vérocuronium
Side effects	• Tachycardia • Hypotension • Neuromuscular block extended
Posology	• IV: 80-100 mcg/kg, then continuously to 100 mcg/kg/h
Method of administration	• Intravenous (IV)

Memo 82

Ipratropium bromide

DCI and name	Ipratropium bromide (Atrovent®)
Pharmacological Class	Anticholinergic bronchodilator by inhalation
Indications	Crisis of asthma, bronchospasm in association with salbutamol
Contra-indications	Known hypersensitivity to one of the components
Side effects	• Dry mouth • Pharyngeal irritation
Posology	Nebulization: - < 20 kg: 0.25 mg/aerosol - > 20 kg: 0.5 mg
Method of administration	Nebulization (aerosol)

Memo

Cefotaxime

DCI and name	Cefotaxime (CLAFORAN®)
Pharmacological Class	Bêtalactamine: 3rd generation cephalosporin
Indications	Severe infection (sepsis, endocardites, meningitis, purpura fulminans)
Contra-indications	Allergy to antibiotics of the Group of cephalosporins
Side effects	• Anaphylactic Reactions • Cutaneous manifestations (rash, pruritus) • Diarrhea • Veinite
Posology	IV: 50 mg/kg (meningeal dose: 100 mg/kg) every 8 h
Method of administration	Intravenous (IV)

Memo

Ceftriaxone

DCI and name	Ceftriaxone (ROCÉPHINE®)
Pharmacological Class	Antibiotic, 3rd generation cephalosporin
Indications	Used in the case of bacterial meningitis or of pyelonephritis
Contra-indications	• Allergy to the group of cephalosporins • New-born premature and
Side effects	• Allergic Rash • Pruritus • Urticaria • Diarrhea • Nausea
Posology	IV/IM: 50 mg/kg (meningeal dose: 100 mg/kg)
Method of administration	• Intravenous (IV) • Intramuscular (IM)

Memo

Activated Charcoal

DCI and name	Activated charcoal (TOXICARB®)
Pharmacological Class	Adsorbent of toxic substances, is opposed to their digestive absorption
Indications	Poisoning and drug overdose, while the substances in question may be present in the digestive tract. Consider the administration of activated charcoal if ingestion < 1 h and if the state of consciousness allows
Contra-indications	Drug therapy > 1 h, disorders of the Conscience, poisoning by caustic products/corrosive
Side effects	Nausea
Posology	PO: 1 g/kg
Method of administration	Per os (PO)

Memo

Clonazepam

DCI and name	Clonazepam (RIVOTRIL®)
Pharmacological Class	Antiepileptics of the class of drugs known as benzodiazepines
Indications	Seizures
Contra-indications	• Known hypersensitivity to the Clonazepam and benzodiazepines • Severe Respiratory Insufficiency • Hepatic insufficiency • Myasthenia gravis • Syndrome of Lennox-Gastaut
Side effects	• Allergies • Disorders of the Conscience • Muscle hypotonia • Nygstagmus
Posology	IV: 0.05-0.1 mg/kg, then 0.1 mg/kg/6 h Duration of action: 6-8 h
Method of administration	Intravenous (IV)

Memo 87
Anesthésiante cream

DCI	Lidocaine, Prilocaine (EMLA 5%)
Pharmacological Class	Local anesthetic, amides
Indications	Anesthesia of the skin during invasive care (installation of track peripheral venous, blood sampling, lumbar puncture, surgical procedure superficially) in association with other painkillers means: Solution Sweet, nitrous oxide
Contra-indications	• Hypersensitivity to lidocaine and/or prilocaine • Porphyria • Congenital methaemoglobinaemia • Do not put cream anesthésiante near the eyes, on the mucous membranes or on of the lesions of eczema
Side effects	• Erythema • Local pallor • Rare purpuriques lesions and the risk of methemoglobinemia in premature infants

Posology	**Recommendation: Premature between 30 and 37 weeks:** a hazelnut (0.5 g) on a single site once a day, one hour maximum of install (outside AMM)

Age	Posology	Application Time
New-born babies and infants 0-2 months	1 g	1 h
Infants 3-11 months	2 g	1 h
Young Children And children 1-5 years	10 g	1-5 h
Children 6-11 years	20 g	1-5 h

Method of administration	• Tube or patch in the skin • Apply the cream in thick layer without spread (hazelnut) and cover it with an adhesive bandage of type " TEGADERM® ". If available, use directly the anaesthetic patch already packaged • Always note the time to install • Wipe off the cream before the CARE

Memo

Diazepam

DCI and name	**Diazepam (Valium®)**
Pharmacological Class	Anxiolytic of the class of drugs known as benzodiazepines
Indications	The first line of treatment used in the convulsive crisis
Contra-indications	• Hypersensitivity to the active principle • Severe Respiratory Insufficiency • Hepatic insufficiency • Myasthenia gravis • Syndrome of Lennox-Gastaut
Side effects	• Anterograde amnesia • Behavior Disorders • Decline of the Vigilance • Drowsiness • Muscle hypotonia • Diplopia
Posology	• IR: 0.5 mg/kg

	• IV: 0.3-0.5 mg/kg
Method of administration	• Intrarectal (IR) • Intravenous (IV)

Memo 89

Dobutamine

DCI and name	Dobutamine (DOBUTREX®)
Pharmacological Class	Adrenergic and dopaminergic therapy
Indications	Low flow, state of shock (at best guided by the ultrasound)
Contra-indications	• Mechanical barrier for filling or the ejection (ventricular obstructive cardiomyopathy, Aortic valvular disease, patients with obstruction dynamic intraventricularly) • Hypersensitivity to dobutrex
Side effects	• Increase of heart rate • Increase in blood pressure
Posology	IV: 5-20 mcg/kg/min Attention: inactivation by bicarbonate
Method of administration	• Intravenous (IV)

Memo

Dopamine

DCI	Dopamine
Pharmacological Class	Adrenergic and dopaminergic therapy
Indications	• Syndrome of low flow • State of Shock • Significant Hypotension (used in Neonatal)
Contra-indications	• Mechanical barrier for filling or the ejection • Hypersensitivity to dopamine
Side effects	• Disorders of the rhythm • Nausea • Vomiting
Posology	IV: 5 to 10 mcg/kg/min Attention: inactivation by bicarbonate
Method of administration	Intravenous (IV)

Memo

Esomeprazole

DCI and name	Esomeprazole (INEXIUM®)
Pharmacological Class	Proton Pump Inhibitors
Indications	• Gastro-esophageal • Peptic ulcers • Digestive bleeding
Contra-indications	Known hypersensitivity to the active substance or to any of the components
Side effects	• Diarrhea • Headache
Posology	• PO: 1-2 mg/kg/i • IV: 1 mg/kg/I on 10 to 30 min
Method of administration	Per os (PO)

Memo

Etomidate

DCI and name	Etomidate (HYPNOMIDATE®)
Pharmacological Class	General Anaesthetic
Indications	• Hypnotic to short duration of action used in the induction • AMM: > 2 years
Contra-indications	• Adrenal insufficiency • To avoid when Sepsis • Known hypersensitivity to the active substance or to any of the components
Side effects	• Dyskinesia • Myoclonus • Rash
Posology	IV: 0.2-0.4 mg/kg Time limit for action: 30 s Duration of action: 5-10 min
Method of administration	Intravenous (IV)

Memo 93
Fentanyl

DCI	Fentanyl
Pharmacological Class	Morphinomimétique
Indications	Central analgesic reserved for anesthesia of short, medium and long duration
Contra-indications	• Known hypersensitivity to fentanyl • Respiratory depression not assisted, association to the AGONISTS-ANTAGONISTS (nalbuphine, buprenorphine, pentazocine)
Side effects	• Respiratory Depression • Apnea • Bradycardia • Hypotension • Myoclonus • Nausea • Vomiting
Posology	IV:

	- Loading dose : 3-4 mcg/kg
	- Maintenance: 1-4 mcg/kg/h
	Time limit for action: 2-3 min
	Duration of action: 20 to 30 min
Method of administration	Intravenous (IV)

Memo

Flumazenil

DCI and name	Flumazenil (ANEXATE®)
Pharmacological Class	Antidote imidazo-benzodiazepine
Indications	The antagonists of benzodiazepines and related molecules
Contra-indications	In case of hypersensitivity or intolerance known to this product
Side effects	• Nausea • Vomiting • Anxiety • Palpitations
Posology	• IV: 10 mcg/kg (max. 2 mg), can be repeated every 60 s (max. 4 times) • In continuous: 10 mcg/kg/h
Method of administration	Intravenous (IV)

Memo

Fosphenytoin

DCI and name	Fosphenytoin (PRODILANTIN®)
Pharmacological Class	Antiepileptics
Indications	Status epilepticus
Contra-indications	• Hypersensitivity to the fosphenytoin sodium or to the excipients of the product • Deficit in G6PD • Hepatic insufficiency • Porphyries • AMM > 5 years
Side effects	• Cardiovascular collapse • Disorders of the conduction (QT prolongation) • Hypotension • Nygstagmus • Dizziness • Headache • Drowsiness

Posology	IVL: dose of load: 15-20 mg/kg (under Recording Continuous ECG) Maintenance: 3-8 mg/kg/24 h to divide into 3 IVL Deadline for action: 15-25 min
Method of administration	• Intravenous (IV)

Memo

Furosemide

DCI and name	Furosemide (Lasilix®)
Pharmacological Class	Diuretic
Indications	• Sodium Retention severe cardiac origin, renal, cirrhotic • Emergencies cardiac: acute edema of the lung
Contra-indications	• Hypersensitivity to furosemide or to any of the excipients • Acute renal failure functional • Hepatic Encephalopathy • Obstruction on the urinary tract • Hypovolemia or dehydration • Severe hypokalemia • Severe hyponatremia • Hepatitis in evolution and insufficient severe hepatocellular
Side effects	• Hypotension • Fluid and Electrolyte Disturbance

	• Dehydration • Hypovolemia
Posology	IV: 1 mg/kg/8-12 h
Method of administration	Intravenous (IV)

Memo

Gentamicin

DCI	Gentamicin
Pharmacological Class	Antibacterial antibiotic of the family of the aminoglycosides
Indications	In association with the ßlactamines for the maternal infections fetal-
Contra-indications	Allergy to antibiotics of the family of the aminoglycosides
Side effects	• Ototoxicity • Renal Insufficiency (in the case of overdose, extended treatment, renal impairment earlier)
Posology	• IV new-born: | Post Age-conceptionnel	< 30 SA	30-33 its	34-36 its	≥ 37 its
---	---	---	---	---
Posology	7 mg/kg	6.5 mg/kg	6 mg/kg	5.5 mg/kg	 Spacing of doses in function of the term

	• **IV child:** 5 mg/kg on 20 min/24 h
Method of administration	Intravenous (IV)

Memo 98
Glucagon

DCI and name	Glucagon (GLUCAGEN®)
Pharmacological Class	The glycogenolytic hormones, hyperglycémiante substance which mobilizes the hepatic glycogen
Indications	Severe hypoglycaemia
Contra-indications	Hypersensitivity to glucagon or lactose
Side effects	• Nausea • Vomiting • Abdominal Pain
Posology	IM: - Among the child > 25 kg = 1 mg - Among the child < 25 kg = 0.5 mg
Method of administration	Intramuscular (IM)

Hemisuccinate of hydrocortisone

DCI and name	**Hemisuccinate of hydrocortisone (hydrocortisone®)**
Pharmacological Class	Glucocorticoid hormone
Indications	• Substitution treatment in the course of the adrenal insufficiency • Hypotension of premature (opinion neonatologist)
Contra-indications	The counter-usual indications of the General corticosteroid do not apply to doses recommended proxy
Side effects	Neurocognitive retinal and in the long term in the premature
Posology	• **New-born:** 0.5 mg to 1 mg/kg every 6 h • **Child:** indication of the adrenal insufficiency acute: 5 mg/kg
Method of administration	Intravenous (IV)

Memo

Hydroxocobalamine

DCI and name	Hydroxocobalamine (CYANOKIT®)
Pharmacological Class	Antidote
Indications	Intoxications by cyanide by the smoke of fire
Contra-indications	No
Side effects	Red coloration of the skin and urine
Posology	IV: 70 mg/kg in 15 min
Method of administration	Intravenous (IV)

Hydroxyzine

DCI and name	Hydroxyzine (Atarax®)
Pharmacological Class	Anxiolytic
Indications	Antihistamine, premedication, minor manifestations of anxiety, symptomatic treatment of hives
Contra-indications	• Patient presenting an elongation acquired congenital or known to the QT interval • Allergy to any of the components
Side effects	• Drowsiness • Headache • Fatigue • Dry mouth
Posology	PO: 1 mg/kg/I in 1 to 2 times
Method of administration	Per os (PO)

Memo

Ibuprofen

DCI	Ibuprofen
Pharmacological Class	Non-steroidal anti-inflammatory drug
Indications	• Pain
	• Anti-inflammatory property
	• Treatment of fever (second intent)
Contra-indications	• Hypersensitivity to ibuprofen
	• History of hemorrhage
	• Ulcer
	• Severe hepatic impairment
	• Severe heart failure
	• Renal failure
	• Chickenpox
Side effects	• Digestive Disorders
	• Dermatologic Reactions
Posology	PO: 10 mg/kg/8 h
Method of administration	Per os (PO)

Memo 103

Insulin

DCI and name	Insulin (Actrapid®, UMULINE®)
Pharmacological Class	Insulins and analogues for injection, quick action, insulin human
Indications	Fast-acting insulin
Contra-indications	Hypersensitivity to the active principle
Side effects	• Hypoglycemia • Edema • Reactions at the injection site
Posology	IV: 0.05 IU/kg/h (max. 0.1 IU/kg/h) in continuous IV
Method of administration	Intravenous (IV)

Memo 104
Ketamine

DCI and name	Ketamine (KÉTALAR®)
Pharmacological Class	General Anaesthetic
Indications	Anesthesia and induction of the status asthmaticus
Contra-indications	• Recognized hypersensitivity to ketamine • Severe heart failure • Severe Hypertension
Side effects	• Increase in heart rate and blood pressure • Respiratory depression moderate apnea or • Diplopia or nystagmus • Hallucinations
Posology	• Induction IV: 2-4 mg/kg • Sedation/analgesia IV: 0.2-0.5 mg/kg • IR: 5-10 mg/kg • Time of action: 60 s

	• Duration of action: 5-15 min
Method of administration	• Intravenous (IV) • Intrarectal (IR)

Memo

Mannitol 10%

DCI	Mannitol 10%
Pharmacological Class	Carbohydrate practically non-metabolizable producing osmotic diuresis
Indications	• Cerebral edema • Intracranial hypertension
Contra-indications	• Hyperosmolarité preexisting plasma • Dehydration • Congestive Heart Failure
Side effects	• Electrolyte imbalance • Nausea • Vomiting • Headache • Dizziness • Acute renal failure
Posology	IV: 0.5-1 g/kg in 15 min
Method of administration	Intravenous (IV)

Memo 106
Methylprednisolone

DCI and name	Methylprednisolone (SOLUMÉDROL®)
Pharmacological Class	Glucocorticoid anti-inflammatory steroidal
Indications	• Corticosteroids • Treatment of the Angiedema • Anaphylactic Shock • Cerebral edema • Laryngeal dyspnea • Acute Asthma serious
Contra-indications	Some viral diseases in Evolution (hepatitis, herpes, chicken pox, herpes zoster)
Side effects	• Euphoria • Excitement • Rare cases of anaphylaxis
Posology	IV: 1-2 mg/kg
Method of administration	Intravenous (IV)

Metronidazole

DCI and name	Metronidazole (Flagyl®)
Pharmacological Class	Antibacterial antibiotics, pest control of the family of nitro-5-imidazole
Indications	Ulcéro enterocolitis necrotizing- (ECUN) of premature
Contra-indications	• Hypersensitivity to metronidazole or of the family of imidazole • Wheat allergy
Side effects	• Digestive disorders Mild • Allergy (pruritus) • Headache • Dizziness
Posology	• **IV new-born** - If < 40 Its → 15 mg/kg/ 12 h - 40 Its to J7 → 15 mg/kg/ 8 h • **IV child:** 20 to 30 mg/kg/I in 3 times
Method of administration	Intravenous (IV)

Memo

Midazolam

DCI and name	Midazolam (HYPNOVEL®)
Pharmacological Class	Hypnotic and sedative to quick action, derived from benzodiazepines
Indications	• Sedation Vigil • Anesthesia • Anticonvulsant
Contra-indications	Known hypersensitivity to benzodiazepines
Side effects	• Hypotension • Bradycardia • Decrease in vigilance • Drowsiness • Headache
Posology	• Intrajugal (the active principle of BUCCOLAM®): 0.3 mg/kg • IV: 50-100 mcg/kg • IV continues: - Premature = 30 mcg/kg/h

	- Child = 50-100 mcg/kg/h
	Time limit for action: 2-3 min
	Duration of action: 10-20 min
	Intranasal •: 0.3 mg/kg (deadline for action: 5-10 min)
Method of administration	• Intrajugal Intravenous •

Memo

Morphine

DCI	Morphine
Pharmacological Class	Opioid Analgesics
Indications	Intense pain or rebels to painkillers of Level I and II
Contra-indications	• Hypersensitivity to morphine or to the other constituents • Respiratory Insufficiency • Inadequate severe hepatocellular • Epilepsy not controlled • Associations with buprenorphine, nalbuphine and pentazocine
Side effects	• Drowsiness • Confusion • Nausea • Vomiting • Constipation • Respiratory distress • Dysuria or urinary retention

Posology	• IV: dose of load: 50-100 mcg/kg, then 25 mcg/kg in titration • Maintenance: 20-40 mcg/kg/h
Method of administration	Intravenous (IV)

Memo

N-acetyl-cysteine

DCI and name	N-acetyl-cysteine (FLUIMUCIL®)
Pharmacological Class	Amino acid derivative
Indications	Used as an antidote to the paracetamol
Contra-indications	History of hypersensitivity to any of the components
Side effects	• Risk of bronchial surencombrement, particularly in infants and in some patients unable to effective sputum • Skin reactions allergic to such as pruritus, erythematous rash, urticaria and angiedema
Posology	N-acetyl-cysteine should be started less than 8 h post-ingestion. If it is not possible to obtain a metering before this period, administer the antidote. If a dosage is available (reliable if fact ≥ 4 h post-ingestion), refer to the nomogram of Rumack.

Doses	Children	Children	Children

	< 20 kg	20-40 kg	> 40 kg
Loading dose 150 mg/kg IV in 15 min	In 3 ml/kg of G5%	In 100 ml of G5%	In 200 ml of G5%
Then 50 mg/kg IV in 4 h	In 7 ml/kg of G5%	In 250 ml of G5%	In 500 ml of G5%
Then 100 mg/kg IV in 16 h	In 14 ml/kg of G5%	In 500 ml of G5%	In 1 000 ml of G5%
Slow down or stop the infusion rate if anaphylactic reaction Mild or severe			
Method of administration	Intravenous (IV)		

Memo

Nalbuphine

DCI and name	Nalbuphine (NUBAIN®)
Pharmacological Class	Central analgesic semi-synthetic type/agonist morphine antagonist of the series of phenanthrenes
Indications	• Pain, install thoracic drain in the child • AMM: > 18 months
Contra-indications	Hypersensitivity to the nalbuphine, association to morphinomimétiques, Pure Agonists
Side effects	• Drowsiness • Dizziness • Nausea • Vomiting • Sweating • Dry mouth • Headache
Posology	• IV: 0.2 mg/kg/4 h or 1.2 mg/kg/i in IV continues

	Time limit for action: 2-3 min
	• IR: 400 mcg/kg or 0.4 mg/kg
	Time limit for action: 10-15 min
Method of administration	• Intravenous (IV) • Intrarectal (IR)

Memo

Naloxone

DCI and name	Naloxone (Narcan®)
Pharmacological Class	Antagonists of Opioids
Indications	• Antidote of Opioids • Differential Diagnosis of toxic comas
Contra-indications	Hypersensitivity to the naloxone
Side effects	• Chills • Hyperventilation • Vomiting • Agitation
Posology	• IV: 10 mcg/kg all 2-3 min • In continuous: 10 mcg/kg/h
Method of administration	Intravenous (IV)

Memo

Néfopam

DCI and name	Néfopam (ACUPAN®)
Pharmacological Class	Central analgesic non-opioid
Indications	Symptomatic treatment of disorders Acute painful
Contra-indications	Child of less than 15 years
Side effects	• Drowsiness • Nausea
Posology	IV or IM: 20 mg
Method of administration	• Intravenous (IV) • Intramuscular (IM)

Memo

Nicardipine

DCI and name	Nicardipine (LOXEN®)
Pharmacological Class	Antihypertensive agent IV, Calcium Channel Blockers
Indications	High blood pressure
Contra-indications	Known hypersensitivity to the nicarpidine
Side effects	• Edema of the lower limbs • Headache • Flushing • Palpitations • Dizziness
Posology	• IV: 0.5-3 mcg/kg/min • Loading dose: 10 to 20 mcg/kg if vital emergency
Method of administration	Intravenous (IV)

Noradrenaline

DCI and name	Noradrenaline (LEVOPHED®)
Pharmacological Class	Sympathomimetic
Indications	Emergency treatment of collapse and for the restoration and maintenance of the blood pressure, during or at the end of the 2e filling
Contra-indications	No
Side effects	• Skin necrosis in the event of extravasation • Anxiety • Respiratory discomfort • Headache • Retrosternal pain or pharyngeal • Vomiting
Posology	Start at 0.1 mcg/kg/min, continuous infusion and then titration
Method of administration	Intravenous (IV)

Memo 116
Ondansetron

DCI and name	Ondansetron (Zophren®)
Pharmacological Class	• Antagonist of serotonin • Antiemetics, 5-HT3 Receptor Antagonists
Indications	The prevention of acute nausea and vomiting
Contra-indications	Hypersensitivity to ondansetron or to any of the excipients
Side effects	• Allergy • Headache • Puff of heat • Flush • Constipation
Posology	IV: - < 10 kg: 2 mg - ≤ 6 years: 4 mg - ≥ 6 years: 8 mg
Method of	Intravenous (IV)

| administration | |

Memo

Paracetamol

DCI and name	Paracetamol (PERFALGAN®)
Pharmacological Class	Analgesic and antipyretic drug
Indications	• Treatment of pain of moderate intensity and of the hyperthermia
Contra-indications	• Hypersensitivity to paracetamol • Inadequate severe hepatocellular
Side effects	• Malaise • Hypotension • Reaction at the site of injection
Posology	• IV: 15 mg/kg • PO: 15 mg/kg/6 h • New-born: - 28-31 ITS: 10 mg/kg/12 h > - 31 Its: 10 mg/kg/6 h > - 41 ITS and 3 weeks of life: 15 mg/kg/6 h
Method of administration	• Intravenous (IV) • Per os (PO)

Memo 118
Phenobarbital

DCI and name	Phenobarbital (GARDÉNAL®)
Pharmacological Class	Barbiturate
Indications	Status epilepticus
Contra-indications	• Porphyries • Hypersensitivity to barbiturates • Syndrome of Dravet
Side effects	• Drowsiness • Depressant effect cardiovascular and sedative potentiated by benzodiazepines
Posology	IV: - **New-born:** 20 mg/kg in 20 min - **Child:** 15 mg/kg in 20 min Dilution physiological serum Time limit for action: 20 min
Method of administration	Intravenous (IV)

Memo

Phenytoin

DCI and name	Phenytoin (DILANTIN®)
Pharmacological Class	Anticonvulsant
Indications	Status epilepticus
Contra-indications	• Hypersensitivity to any of the components • Deficit in G6PD • Hepatic insufficiency • Porphyries
Side effects	• Cardiovascular collapse and/or depression of the central nervous system • Disorders of the PACE and the conduction (QT prolongation) • Tissue necrosis in the event of extravasation
Posology	• IV: 15 mg/kg in 20 min (dilute with the physiological serum and infuse to hand, the risk of precipitation)

	Under Recording Continuous ECG
	Time limit for action: 6 to 10 min
	Duration of action: 8 to 10 h
Method of administration	Intravenous (IV)

Memo

Propofol

DCI and name	Propofol (DIPRIVAN®)
Pharmacological Class	General Anesthetics
Indications	Anaesthetic of quick action to use at the time of the Induction
Contra-indications	• Known hypersensitivity to propofol • Arterial Hypotension • Hemodynamic instability
Side effects	• Hypotension, which may be severe • Bradycardia • Greasy embolism • Always < 48 h and < 5 mg/kg/h = RISK OF taken: syndrome of infusion of propofol potentially fatal, rhabdomyolise, heart failure, arrhythmia, metabolic acidosis, hyperlipidemia, myoglobinuria
Posology	IV: - 2-4 mg/kg

	- New-born: 1 mg/kg before intubation with stable hemodynamic
Method of administration	Intravenous (IV)

Memo

Propranolol

DCI and name	**Propranolol (AVLOCARDYL®)**
Pharmacological Class	Beta-blocking
Indications	Malaise of the tetralogy of Fallot (in association with the Valium)
Contra-indications	• Chronic Obstructive Pulmonary Disease • Cardiogenic shock • Hypotension
Side effects	• Asthenia • Bradycardia
Posology	IV: 1 mg IVL diluted in 4 ml of G5% or physiological serum to move slowly up to Decrease in heart rate and recurrence of breath
Method of administration	Intravenous (IV)

Memo

Nitrous oxide

DCI and name	Nitrous oxide (MEOPA®)
Pharmacological Class	Equimolar mixture oxygen (50%), nitrous oxide (50%) and colorless and odorless gas
Indications	• Anxiolytic and analgesia surface, to use in association with cream anesthésiante, methods of distraction and/or other treatment for pain • Any painful act of short duration
Contra-indications	• Head trauma, intracranial hypertension • Alteration of the state of consciousness • Pneumothorax • Bubble of emphysema • Gaseous embolism • Abdominal distension, PNEUMOPERITONEUM • Facial Trauma

	• Known deficit and not substituted for vitamin B12
Side effects	• Nausea, vomiting • Dysphoria • Anguish • Malaise
Posology	• To breathe the gas 3 min to the child for that it begins to act • Continue the inhalation during the entire duration of the Act • The balloon present on the system of inhalation should never be collabé, it must always adapt the gas flow
Method of administration	Inhalation gas

Salbutamol

DCI and name	Salbutamol (Ventolin®)
Pharmacological Class	Bronchodilator beta-2 mimetic of short duration to quick action
Indications	Treatment of Asthma
Contra-indications	Allergy to one of the components
Side effects	• Sinus tachycardia • Heart Rhythm Disorders • Digestive Disorders • Skin allergy • Dizziness
Posology	• Spray: 1 puff/3 kg (min. 2/max. 10) • Nebulization: - < 20 kg: 2.5 mg - > 20 kg: 5 mg • Continuous nebulization: 0.45 mg/kg/h • IV: 0,5-5 mcg/kg/min (5 mcg/kg in the case of chest blocked)

Method of administration	• Inhalation (spray, nebulization) • Intravenous (IV)

Memo 124

Salted serum hypertonic NaCl 7.5%

DCI	Salted serum hypertonic NaCl 7.5%
Pharmacological Class	The solutes crystalloids
Indications	• Cerebral edema • Intracranial hypertension • Cranial Trauma with hypovolemic shock
Contra-indications	Congestive Heart Failure
Side effects	Ionic disorders (hyperchloraemic acidosis)
Posology	IV: 3 ml/kg in 5-10 min
Method of administration	Intravenous (IV)

Memo

Sweet solution to Referred Pain Reliever

DCI and name	Sucrose solution 24% (ALGOPEDOL®)
Indications	• In the newborn and the infant up to 4-6 months • Referred pain reliever associated to the suction not nutritious, to care containers, to the Cream anesthésiante • To use when invasive care (installation of track, venous blood sample, installing gastric probe, bandage...) or of discomfort (nursing) • Breastfeeding produces the same effect
Contra-indications	• Atresia of the esophagus, oesotrachéale fistula not operated • Known intolerance to fructose • Enterocolitis • Swallowing Disorders

Side effects	Desaturation and risk of false route if the administration too fast especially in the premature The administration of sugar solution does not alter the blood glucose levels!	
Posology	Weight	Posology
	< 1 000 g	1 to 2 drops (0.05 to 0.1 ml)
	Of 1 000 g to 1 500 g	3 to 4 drops (0.15 to 0.2 ml)
	Of 1 500 g to 2 000 g	5 to 7 drops (0.25 to 0.35 ml)
	≥ 2 000 g	8 to 10 drops (0.4 to 0.5 ml)
	Maximum 6 to 8 times per day	
Method of administration	• Per os (PO): Administer on the language, drip, using a syringe • The analgesic effect appears 1-2 min after the administration and has a duration of action of 5-7	

| | min |
| | • Renew the administration if the care lasts for more than 5 min |

Memo

Sufentanil

DCI	Sufentanil
Pharmacological Class	Opioid anesthetic
Indications	Central analgesic reserved for anesthesia-intensive care
Contra-indications	Known hypersensitivity to the sufentanil, association to the agonists/antagonists Opioids
Side effects	• Pruritus • Nausea • Vomiting • Constipation • Globe Of The Bladder • Respiratory distress
Posology	IV: in dose of load: 0.2-0.3 mcg/kg Continuous: 0.2-0.3 mcg/kg/h Time limit for action: 1-2 min Duration of action: 50-70 min
Method of	Intravenous (IV)

administration	

Memo

Magnesium Sulfate

DCI	Magnesium Sulfate
Pharmacological Class	The electrolytes
Indications	• Athmes serious acute • Curative treatment of torsades de pointes • Acute Hypokaliémies • Intakes magnesians
Contra-indications	Severe renal impairment
Side effects	• Pain at the point of injection • Vasodilation with sensation of heat
Posology	IV: 25-40 mg/kg in 20 min, under control continuous ECG
Method of administration	Intravenous (IV)

Memo 128

Morphine sulfate

DCI and name	Morphine sulphate **(ORAMORPH®)**
Pharmacological Class	Opioid analgesic. Oral morphine to immediate release
Indications	Intense pain or rebels to painkillers of Level I and II.
Contra-indications	• Hypersensitivity to morphine or to the other constituents • Respiratory Insufficiency • Inadequate severe hepatocellular • Epilepsy not controlled • Associations with buprenorphine, nalbuphine and pentazocine
Side effects	• Drowsiness • Confusion • Nausea • Vomiting • Constipation • Respiratory distress

	• Dysuria or urinary retention
Posology	Single-dose container of 10 mg/5 ml PO: 1 mg/kg/day Max dose: 20 mg > 5 kg = 0.5 mg/kg in dose of load and then titration of 0.2 mg/kg/30 min up to effectiveness and then equivalent to the total dose received by titration (without the dose of load)/4 h
Method of administration	Per os (drops)

Memo

Suxaméthonium

DCI and name	Suxaméthonium (CÉLOCURINE®)
Pharmacological Class	Peripherally acting muscle relaxant
Indications	Curare to cause a muscular relaxation of short duration, used for the endotracheal intubation
Contra-indications	• Allergy to any of the components • Neuromuscular Disease • Myopathy • Hyperkalemia • Burned > 48 h • Denervation, > 48 h
Side effects	• Anaphylactic Reaction • Bradycardia • Disorders of the rhythm
Posology	• IV: - < 18 months: 2 mg/kg - > 18 months: 1 mg/kg Deadline for action: 30 to 60 s

	Duration of action: 5 to 10 min
Method of administration	Intravenous (IV)

Memo — Terbutaline

DCI and name	Terbutaline (Bricanyl®)
Pharmacological Class	Bronchodilators beta-2 mimics to delayed action and long-term by the oral route
Indications	Crisis of asthma
Contra-indications	Hypersensitivity to any of the Constituents
Side effects	• Tremor of the extremities • Cramps • Headache
Posology	• Nebulization: 1 drop/kg (min. 8 DROPS // max. 1 Pod 2 ml = 5 mg)
Method of administration	Nebulization (aerosol)

Memo

Thiopental

DCI and names	Thiopental (NESDONAL®, pentothal®)
Pharmacological Class	Intravenous Anesthetic, barbiturate of quick action
Indications	• Induction and maintenance of general anesthesia Intravenous (alone or in combination) • Outbreaks of intracranial hypertension
Contra-indications	• Respiratory obstruction • Acute Asthma serious, status asthmaticus • Porphyria • Hypersensitivity to barbiturates • Immunosuppression
Side effects	• Hypersensitivity including anaphylactic shock • Coughing, sneezing, broncho-laryngospasm in particular during the induction period

	• Arterial Hypotension
	• Cardiac Arrhythmia
	• Respiratory Depression
	• Dizziness
	• Confusion
	• Headache
	• Immunosuppression
	• A decrease of cerebral blood flow that can be deleterious in some epilepsy
	• Tissue necrosis in the event of extravasation
Posology	IV: 5 mg/kg, then 1-3 mg/kg/h (dilute with the physiological serum, to infuse alone, precipitates)
Method of administration	Intravenous (IV)

Memo 132

Tramadol

DCI	Tramadol
Pharmacological Class	Opioid Analgesics
Indications	• Treatment of moderate pain • AMM: drops per os as soon 3 years, Compressed LP from 12 years, capsule to immediate release from 15 years • No AMM IV among the child
Contra-indications	• Known hypersensitivity to tramadol or to opiates • Severe Respiratory Insufficiency • Inadequate hepato-cellular
Side effects	• Confusion • Drowsiness • Nausea • Vomiting • A few cases described of Coma with respiratory distress
Posology	PO: 1-2 mg/kg every 6 h (max. 400

	mg/J)
	1 Drop = 2.5 mg
Method of administration	• Per os (PO) • IV only from 15 years

Memo

Vancomycin

DCI	Vancomycin
Pharmacological Class	Antibacterial antibiotic of the family of the glycopeptides
Indications	Infections due to germs sensitive to vancomycin (including staph)
Contra-indications	• Known hypersensitivity to vancomycin • Renal failure
Side effects	• Anaphylactoid Reactions • Nephrotoxicity • Ototoxicity • Nausea • Vomiting
Posology	• **Discontinuous IV IVL in 30 min:** - < 29 Its: 15 mg/kg/i - 30-33 ITS: 15 mg/kg/18 h - 34-37 ITS: 15 mg/kg/12 h - 38-41 ITS: 15 mg/kg/8 h

	- >41 lts: 10 mg/kg/6 h • **IV continuous:** loading dose: 15 mg/kg IVL/30 min, then continuous infusion = - < 37 Sa: 30 mg/kg/i - > 37 Sa: 40 mg/kg/i • **Meningeal reached: 60 mg/kg/i**
Method of administration	Intravenous (IV)

Memo 134

Vitamin K1

DCI	Vitamin K1
Pharmacological Class	An antihaemorrhagic/styptic. Indispensable factor in hepatic synthesis of several factors of the coagulation
Indications	Treatment of prophylaxis of hemorrhagic disease of the Newborn
Contra-indications	History of allergy to vitamin K
Side effects	• Hematoma by track IV • Allergic Reaction
Posology	• IV: 1 mg, or 0.1 ml (whatever the weight) • PO: 2 mg
Method of administration	• Intravenous (IV) • Per os (PO)

Part 5

Legislation

>>> Mémo 135 - Accident d'exposition au sang (AES)

>>> Mémo 136 - Certificats

>>> Mémo 137 - Décret Ambulancier

>>> Mémo 138 - Hémovigilance

>>> Mémo 139 - Matériovigilance

>>> Mémo 140 - Pharmacovigilance

Memo 135
Accident of exposure to blood (AES)

I ♦ Definition
The accident of exposure to blood (AES) is defined by a percutaneous contact (pricking, cuts) or mucosal (eye, mouth) with blood or a biological product. He exposes to the risk of bacterial contamination and/or viral.
This type of accident concerns the whole of the personal on intervention, and it is increased by the number and speed of the actions implemented within a environment sometimes unfavorable.

II ♦ measures of prevention systematic
- Port of **gloves** mandatory.
- Port of **mask** to Visor or glasses, if risk of projection.
- Elimination of the waste **as and to the extent** of care (box to needles, garbage).
- Use of systems for collection called " **closed** ".
- **Isolation** of DM reusable.
- Immunization against hepatitis B.

III ♦ conduct to be taken in cases of AES

♦ In case of bite, cut, or contact on skin
- Do not bleed.
- Clean the wound with water and mild soap, liquid, then rinse.
- Disinfect with a solution of _Dakin®_ during 5 minutes.

♦ In case of projection on the mucous membranes
Rinse thoroughly to the physiological serum or in the water for 5 minutes.

♦ On intervention
Search, if possible, the serologic status of the patient (HIV, HCV, HVB) or assessment of risk behaviors.

♦ **return to base**
►Complete the workbook of statement of work accidents.
►Contact, in 4 hours, the referring doctor of the institution or the service of Medicine of work for collection of sérologies +/- prophylactic treatment.

Memo 136
Certificates

I ♦ Definition
A ~~medical~~ certificate is a ~~medical-legal document governed by a legislative text or regulatory. It engages the responsibility of its editor. In préhospitalier, it is essential to have the forms in several copies:~~
- Certificate of Death;
- Certificate of birth;
- Certificate of Birth (normal and child born without life).

II ♦ The Death Certificate
♦ Administrative obligation in accordance with the Decree of 24 December 1996 :

" The authorisation to close the coffin may not be issued that in view of this certificate established by a physician, certifying the death "

(art. L. 2223-42 of the General Code of the territorial communities).
♦ Legal basis of the finding of the death:
- The more important therefore to well the fill that the death is suspect;
- Imperative need to verify the identity of the deceased (and in doubt do not enter anything or put "X"), since deceased declare a living person induces a legal situation Administrative-complex.

♦ Composition
♦ The first three senior slips include:
- The state exact civilian of the deceased;
- Information on the date and the time of death;
- The presence or the absence of an obstacle medico-legal, of obligation in immediate beer, obstacle to the donation of the body or of a pacemaker;
- The request of autopsy;
- The signature and the stamp of the doctor writing the certificate.

These parties are intended to the city hall of the place of establishment of the funerary chamber, to the burial chamber and at the city hall of the place of death.

◆-The 2nd part, bottom, detachable and sealed, is intended to the ARS and then at Inserm. It is strictly confidential and details the circumstances and the cause of death for statistical purposes.

◆ Conditions of drafting

Be registered physician to the order and be present on the spot. The death certificate is writes with the part of the identity of the deceased (mandatory). In the absence of an official document confirming the exact identity of the deceased, the certificate will be drafted under the identity X.

Since a few years, the death certificates electronics are possible. It must be equipped with a computer tool connected and equipped with a printer, so rarely process used in préhospitalier.

III ◆ The birth certificate

◆-The ~~birth certificate~~ is prepared by the doctor or midwife who performed the birth and it is governed by the Articles 56 and 57 of the Civil Code:

" *The birth of the child will be declared by the father, or, in default of the Father, by the doctors in medicine or surgery, midwives, health officers or other persons who will have attended the birth; and when the mother will be born out of his home by the person in the home that she will be mother. The act of birth will be drafted immediately.* "

◆-It must include the following elements:
- The day, time and the exact place of birth;
- The sex of the child;
- The given names, surnames, date of birth and home of the mother;
- The reference to "born viable and living";

- The name of the hospital and of the service in which is transported the new-born;
- The attainment or non-attainment of the issuance (special feature of the préhospitalier);
- The name, signature and stamp of the medical staff the drafting.

IV ♦ The medical certificate of birth

- The ~~medical certificate of birth~~ is used in the case of a child:
- Born without life, regardless of the term (except false early layer ≤ 15 SA or IVG);
- Born Alive and then died if the child is not viable (< 22 ITS and < 500 g).
- It leaves the possibility for parents to give him a name, the register on the Family Booklet and the Bury.

Note. If the child is born alive and viable and then dies, then a birth certificate is normally established as well as a certificate of death of green color, specific for children of less than 28 days.

Memo 137

Ambulance decree

Stopped

Order of 26 April 1999 relating to the formation of adaptation to the employment of drivers ambulance attendants of mobile service of emergency and resuscitation of the public hospital service

NOR: mesh992   1503A

Consolidated version to 12 July 2015

The Secretary of State for Health and Social Action,

Seen the Act No. 86-33 of 9 January 1986 amended the statutory provisions relating to the public hospital service;

Given the Decree No. 91-45 of 14 January 1991 on the Particular Statutes of personal workers, of drivers, conductors, ambulance attendants and of personal maintenance and safety of the public hospital service;

Given the decree n° 97-619 of 30 May 1997 relating to the authorization of mobile services of emergency and resuscitation and modifying the Public Health Code (Second part: Decrees in Council of State), in particular Article R. 712-71-3,

Article 1

The duration of the training of adaptation to the employment of drivers ambulance attendants of the public hospital service affected in a mobile service of emergency and resuscitation is set at four weeks.

Article 2

To be assigned in a mobile service of emergency and resuscitation, the ambulance drivers of the public hospital service must have benefited from the formation of adaptation to employment governed by this order and have carried out, in advance, an internship of road safety and driving in a state of emergency in an approved training center.

Article 3

The training includes four modules described in the Annex and are delivered by the Centers for the teaching of emergency care. The modalities of education are based on the techniques of active pedagogy:

Module 1 : radiotelephone (two days);

Module 2: hygiene, decontamination and disinfection (two days);

Module 3: Situation of exception (two days);

Module 4: participation in the care of a patient within a medical team (nine days).

In the course of the formation of adaptation to employment governed by this Order, an internship of a duration of one week which will be the subject of a report of a course will be conducted in a mobile service of emergency and resuscitation of the interrégion. The list of mobile services of emergency and resuscitation is proposed to the trainees by the Center of Teaching of emergency care.

Article 4

The formation of adaptation to the employment cannot be discontinuous and must take place as soon as the appointment of the ambulance driver of the public hospital service to the mobile service of emergency and resuscitation and, in all cases, before the taking of functions.

This training of employment adjustment is validated by an attestation of follow-up of training courses delivered by the Center for the teaching of emergency care.

Article 5

The Director of hospitals in the Department of Employment and Solidarity is responsible for the execution of this Decree, which will be published in the Official Journal of the French Republic.

Annex

Program of the formation of adaptation to the employment of drivers ambulance attendants of mobile service of emergency and resuscitation of the public hospital service.

Article Annex

MODULE 1

Radiotelephony

The purpose of this module is to give the drivers of ambulance mobile service of emergency and resuscitation the means to use, in an efficient and effective manner, the radiotelephone equipment onboard the vehicle of the mobile service of emergency and resuscitation.

This teaching is carried out in collaboration with the centers of teaching of emergency care providing education leading to the certificate of hospital operator in telecommunications.

Skills to acquire:

Maintain the hardware radio telecommunications in running condition and ensure its proper functioning;

Apply the procedures for the transmission (network health, SSU...);

Use the means of telecommunication; embedded

Identify the different networks and the frequencies used.

MODULE 2

Hygiene, decontamination and disinfection

The purpose of this module is to give drivers affected ambulance within a mobile service of emergency and resuscitation training for the disinfection and decontamination of their vehicle. It includes a theoretical and practical education in the maintenance, disinfection and cleaning of the vehicle, the cell health and some hardware, in the light of the most recent protocols.

Goals to Achieve

At the end of the training, the ambulance driver must be able to:

Apply the rules of hygiene, for itself and its mobile unit hospital, the patient and his entourage and any member of the team;

Apply the principles of decontamination and disinfection of different elements of the health cell;

Apply the various techniques of protection of the patient and the staff on the basis of pathologies encountered ;

Apply the different techniques for the treatment of waste.

MODULE 3

Situation of exception

The purpose of this module is to enable drivers ambulance attendants of EMS to lie in the medical chain of relief and to adapt their behavior to the different situations of exception.

Skills to acquire:

Describe the structures put in place during exceptional situations;

Participate in the implementation and maintenance of the logistics deployed by the Medical Assistance Service urgent and the mobile service of emergency and resuscitation in situation of exception;

Identify the different links in the chain of medical aid;

Apply the rules to be followed by the driver paramedic, in the presence of different situations:
- To the rockshaft ;
- At the Advanced Medical Post;
- To the noria of evacuation;

Participate in the establishment of a mobile PC of transmission and exploit the communication networks.

MODULE 4

Participation in the care of a patient within a medical team

This module allows drivers ambulance mobile service of emergency and resuscitation to adopt the behavior appropriate to each situation and to each patient by performing the preparation of equipment medico-technical and some gestures in the framework of their skills. This module must also enable them to participate in the decision in the psychological burden of the patient and his immediate environment in a situation of medical emergency.

Goals to Achieve

At the end of the training, the ambulance driver must be able to:

Participate in the decision in the overall load of the patient and his entourage.

Apply the methods and the means adapted to the implementation of care and gestures of emergency of the mobile team; hospital

In a medical context or traumatic (among the adult or child):

Identify a neurological distress;

Identify a ventilatory distress;

Identify a circulatory distress;

Participate in the support of a childbirth extrahospitalier unexpectedly;

Participate in the support for a new-born in the framework of transport interhospital;

Participate in the support of a psychiatric emergencies;

Participate in the support of the pain;

Assist in the preparation of the material, on medical prescription;
- Bottles of medical gas and equipment for oxygen therapy;
- Monitoring of the saturation of the OXYGEN - SENSOR INSTALLATION included except in neonatology;
- Assistance in the preparation of the equipment to access; tracheal
- Monitoring expired (Capnography Extension), patient circuit excluded;
- Mechanical ventilator: installation (adjusting parameters and patient circuit excluded);
- Equipment necessary for pleural drainage;
- Monitors électrocardioscopiques, cardiographs, defibrillators in manual mode, coaches électrosystoliques, verification of the electrical load and the recording equipment (installation of electrodes excluded for the defibrillator in manual mode and the Coach électrosystolique);
- Grows-electric syringes;
- Equipment necessary for installing a venous access central or peripheral;
- Installation of the shock trousers (Choice of pressure levels excluded), inflation under control of the physician;
- Monitoring of the non-invasive blood pressure, preparation and implementation;
- Incubator of transport;

Practice within the team of the mobile unit hospitable the gestures of emergency acquired at the end of the teaching of the certificate of capacity paramedic;

Participate in the psychological care of the family and of the entourage;

Know the risks, the signs and the prevention of stress and fatigue professional.

For the Secretary of State and by delegation:

By incapacity of the director of hospitals:

The Deputy Director of Personnel

Of the public hospital service,

D. Vilchien

Memo 138
Haemovigilance

I ♦ Definition
It concerns the blood transfusion chain and allows the reporting of any adverse reaction following the administration of blood products.

II ♦ The device
It is based on three actors:
- **At the national level:** MSNA (National Agency for the safety of the drug and health products);
- **At the regional level:** regional coordinators of haemovigilance (HRC), in collaboration with the ARS;
- **At the local level:** correspondents of haemovigilance.

III ♦ role
Monitor - alert - correct - Prevent

♦ With the transfused patients
Information on the risks of transfusion, monitoring of side effects.

♦ at the level of the traceability of products
National banks of information, labelling of pockets, achievement of patient transfusion allowing to implement link the donor and the recipient.

♦ Reporting of Transfusion accidents
Statement with the sheet of transfusion incident (TIF), a measure of the degree of severity and followed by the MSNA.

IV ♦ security measures in préhospitalier
It is relatively rare to be led to the use of blood products or derivatives in préhospitalier. If this proves to be a necessity, a vehicle (police, VL UAS) will bring on the Places the requested products (PMF more often), via the EFS of the Center hospitalier the closest.

V ♦ The labile blood products

A derivative of the labile blood	Time limits of use	Prétransfusionnelle Security Préhospitalier		
		Levy RAI Group	Crosswalk pocket-EFS sheets	CPU
CGR concentrated red globular	Upon receipt (6 h after receiving between 2°C and 8°C)	X	X	X
CP platelet concentrate	Upon receipt		X	
Pfcs Fresh Frozen Plasma	3 h to max. 6 h after receipt	X	X	
PLY lyophilized plasma (used by the army in the course of the AMM)	- No Time Before Reconstitution - Immediate after reconstitution		X	

VI ♦ The ABO systems

It is defined by the presence or not of antigen (Ag) A and/or B to the surfaces of the RBCS.

- **Group A:** AG has on the surface of the RBCS and Ac anti-B in the plasma.
- ~~Group B:~~ AG B on the surface of the RBCS and Ac anti-A in the plasma.
- **Group O:** No AG has neither B on the surface of the RBCS and Ac anti-A and AC anti-B in the plasma.
- **Group AB:** AG A and B on the surface of the RBCS and not of Ac anti-A or anti-B in the plasma.

♦ **group's respect for transfusions of CGR**

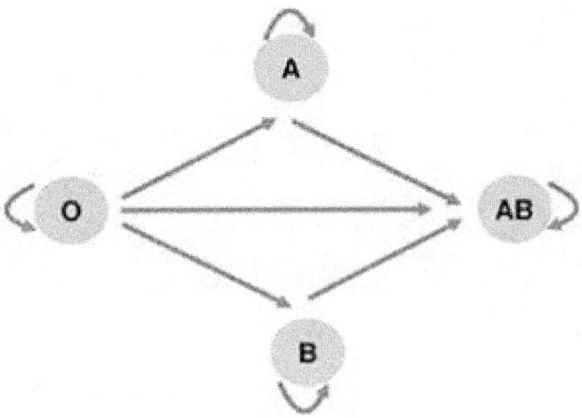

In the context of emergency Pre-hospital, who know neither the Rhesus group of the patient, nor the RAI (research of the presence of agglutinins irregular), only concentrated red globular of group O HR- will be transfused.

♦ group's respect for transfusions of PFCS

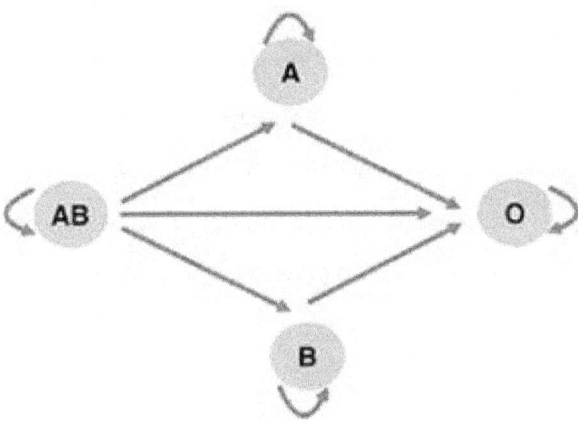

VII ♦ transfusion sheet

Age/weight	Premature < 32 SA and birth weight < 1,500 g	Premature ≥ 32 SA or birth weight ≥ 1 500 g New-born at term Infant
Indication of transfusion (in the absence of hemorrhagic shock)	• Before J7: - Hb < 11 g/dl and ventilatory support with FiO2 ≥ 30% - Hb < 10 g/dl if VS or ventilatory support with FiO2 < 30% • After J7: - Hb < 10 g/dl and	• *If digestive hemorrhage: Hb < 7 g/dl* • If patient traumatized: Strategy to maintain a Hb between 7 and 9 g/dl (outside cranial trauma) • *If cyanotic congenital heart disease: Hb < 12 g/dl* • *Children stabilized in resuscitation under ECMO, or post-operative acute* **of cardiac surgery:** *Hb < 10 g/dl* • Children stabilized in resuscitation without heart disease or in post-op stable correction of heart disease non-cyanogenic: Hb < 8 g/dl • Asymptomatic Anemia and reticulocytes < 100,000/mm3 : Hb < 7 g/dl

	ventilatory support with FiO2 ≥ 30% - ~~Hb <~~ ~~8 g/dl~~ if VS with oxygen or ventilatory support with FiO2 < 30% - ~~Hb < 7 g/dl~~ and reticulocytes < 100 000 mm3 if VS
Type of globular pellet	In the case **of vital emergency** (issuance in the 30 minutes) or **vital emergency immediate** (issuance of the Gall without delay) and absence of given immuno-haematologic of patient: ~~gall o HR- Kel-~~

- Ask for a "**paediatric Preparation**"* If feasible on site.
- ~~Phénotypé~~ HR-KEL1 or extended: all the girls or new-born with maternal RAI.
- ~~Recorded If allo-immunisation feto-maternal (RAI+).~~
- Irradiated in the 6 months following a fetal transfusion or if massive transfusion (except if emergency). Transfusion in 24 h.
- No indication on the CMV negative.

Duration of conservation of Sockets	*• Weight ≤ 1 500 g during the transfusion and volume ≤ 20 ml/kg to the flow rate ≤ 5 ml/kg/h: gall retained ≤ 28 days*	*• If volume ≤ 20 ml/kg to the flow rate ≤ 5 ml/kg/h: gall retained ≤ 42 days*
	• If new-born with instability cardio-respiratory: **gall retained ≤ 14 days**	
	• If Volume > 20 ml/kg (or > 80 ml/kg/i) or flow > 5 ml/kg/h: gall retained ≤ 5 days	
Volume to be transfused	15 ml/kg	20 ml/kg
Modalities of transfusion	On VVP or KTVO	On VVP or central

(Not on épicutanéo catheter-cave)	catheter of large gauge
The gall must be transfused within 6 hours after reception. • *In the absence of bleeding Active: flow rate of 5 ml/kg/h (transfusion on 3 to 4 h).* • *In the presence of a active bleeding: flow rate of 10 ml/kg/h* **on 1 to 2 h.**	
Suspension of the enteral feeding during the transfusion if < 32 ITS and weight < 1 500 g at the time of the transfusion.	
No indication of furosemide.	
Hemorrhagic shock/	• Indication of

Extreme urgency	transfusion: history and clinic or Hb < 6 g/dl
• *Type of globular pellet: gall o HR-Kel-*
• ~~Volume to be transfused: 10 to 20 ml/kg~~ (or more if bleeding is not controlled)
• ~~Terms of transfusion: Begin by serum isotonic salt at the same volume and flow pending~~

~~the globular pellet.~~

Restoration of the hemodynamic: initial bolus of 20 ml On 1 minute. Then flow rate of 10 ml/kg/h.

- ~~Complications to monitor: risk of hyperkalaemia. If massive transfusion: risk of coagulopathy, consider transfusion of PFCS and platelets.~~

* The paediatric preparation is to divide aseptically a PMF in several pediatric units of a minimum volume of 50 ml which can be used either separately or in the framework of a program dedicated to a child. Hemoglobin content is defined in reference to the PMF of origin and the characteristics relating to the aspect, to the hematocrit and the rate of hemolysis are identical to those of the PMF of origin.

Biological data

Neonatal period up to 4 months	After 4 months
ABO group HR Kel	ABO group HR Kel
RAI (red cell antibodies) ~~of the mother~~ between 72 h and prenatal 4 months or postnatal RAI for the child (valid result up to 4 months of age civilian of the Child regardless of the number of transfusions).	RAI collected in the 72 previous h or 21 days if not of immunizing event.
Associate a Antiglobulin testing (direct Coombs) of the child before the first transfusion.	

RAI in reprélever in a period of 1 to 3 months after a transfusion.

Think About It

•Among the child (off premature and infant), the rules of Transfusion in emergency are identical to that of the adult (O HR -)

- Beth Vincent mandatory.
- Do not forget: the traceability, the concordance of the numbers of pockets with the sheet of issuance of EFS, and monitoring during the transfusion even in emergency situations.
- Respect the procedures of your establishment.

Memo 139
Medical Device Vigilance

I ♦ Definition
It concerns the monitoring of any device or medical equipment placed on the market.

Materiovigilance includes the reporting, recording, the assessment and the exploitation of the information reported in a goal of prevention.

Any person falling within a malfunction, an incident or risk of incident by the use of a medical equipment, must establish a Declaration within its establishment through the CLMV.

II ♦ The device
It is based on two main actors:

- At the central level: MSNA (National Agency for the safety of the drug and health products) ;

- At the local level: CLMV (local correspondent of materiovigilance).

III ♦ role of each

♦ **MSNA**
- Records and assesses the risks registered.
- Informs the or the manufacturers concerned by the reports transmitted.
- Request any investigation, including the local correspondents of materiovigilance (CLMV).
- Takes the necessary provisions: animal health measures.

♦ **CLMV (in link with the MSNA)**
- Transmit without delay the serious incidents and quarterly the other.
- Prevents the manufacturers.
- Leads the investigations and the work relating to the safety of DM.
- Ensures locally of the observance of the provisions taken by the MSNA.

♦ **Within its establishment**
•-Stores, analyzes and validates the incidents.
•-Recommends, if necessary, of the precautionary measures.
•-Assistance in reporting.
•-Raises awareness of materiovigilance and to the evaluation of the data.

IV ♦ In Practice
Even in extrahospitalier, any health professional must, in the case of incidents, prevent in a short time his local correspondent (CLMV) of the adverse event in trying to be as specific as possible and keep the evidence (Packaging, Print screen, etc.).

Memo 140

Pharmacovigilance

I ♦ Definition
It aims to guarantee the security of employment of medicines in monitoring their uses, their side effects or undesirable potential or proven.

II ♦ Organization
The ~~pharmacovigilance~~ is organized on the international, national, regional and local level:
- **Local:** via the hospital staff that transmits any undesirable effect in the center of regional reference;
- **Regional:** via the CRPV (regional center of pharmacovigilance) that evaluates and transmits at national level;
- **National:** via the MSNA (National Agency for the safety of the drug and health products) which receives, processes and assesses the alerts. The measures taken are transmitted to the CRPV and then at the hospital level;
- **International:** a network is put in place to ensure that the adverse events observed in some countries can be transmitted to the MSNA.

Pharmaceutical Laboratories must also report directly to the MSNA any serious adverse effect which would be reported. They may also, by a letter to the prescriber, inform health care professionals of a serious adverse reaction.

III ♦ In Practice
Even in extrahospitalier, any health professional must, in the case of an incident, prevent in the shortest possible time his local correspondent (CRPV) of the adverse event (see Mémo 139 " materiovigilance ").

Part 6

The relief plan

>>> Mémo 141 - Plan Orsec Novi

>>> Mémo 142 - Système d'information numérique standardisé (SINUS)

>>> Mémo 143 - SAMU/SMUR

Memo 141

Orsec plan Novi

It is the device implemented on the occasion of a catastrophic accident to limited effect (ACEL) concerning or may involve a large number of victims or of a catastrophic accident with major effects (CMPA).

It is headed by the **commander of relief operations (COS), which has a Director of Fire and Emergency Services (DSIS) and a director of medical relief (DSM)** responsible for the Advanced Medical Post (LDCS) and means of evacuation (UMH, VSAV, PS, ambulances of the Red Cross, civil protection, the Order of Malta and private ambulances if needed).

It is triggered by the prefect.

Here is the diagram of the chain of medical relief in which we will be integrated:

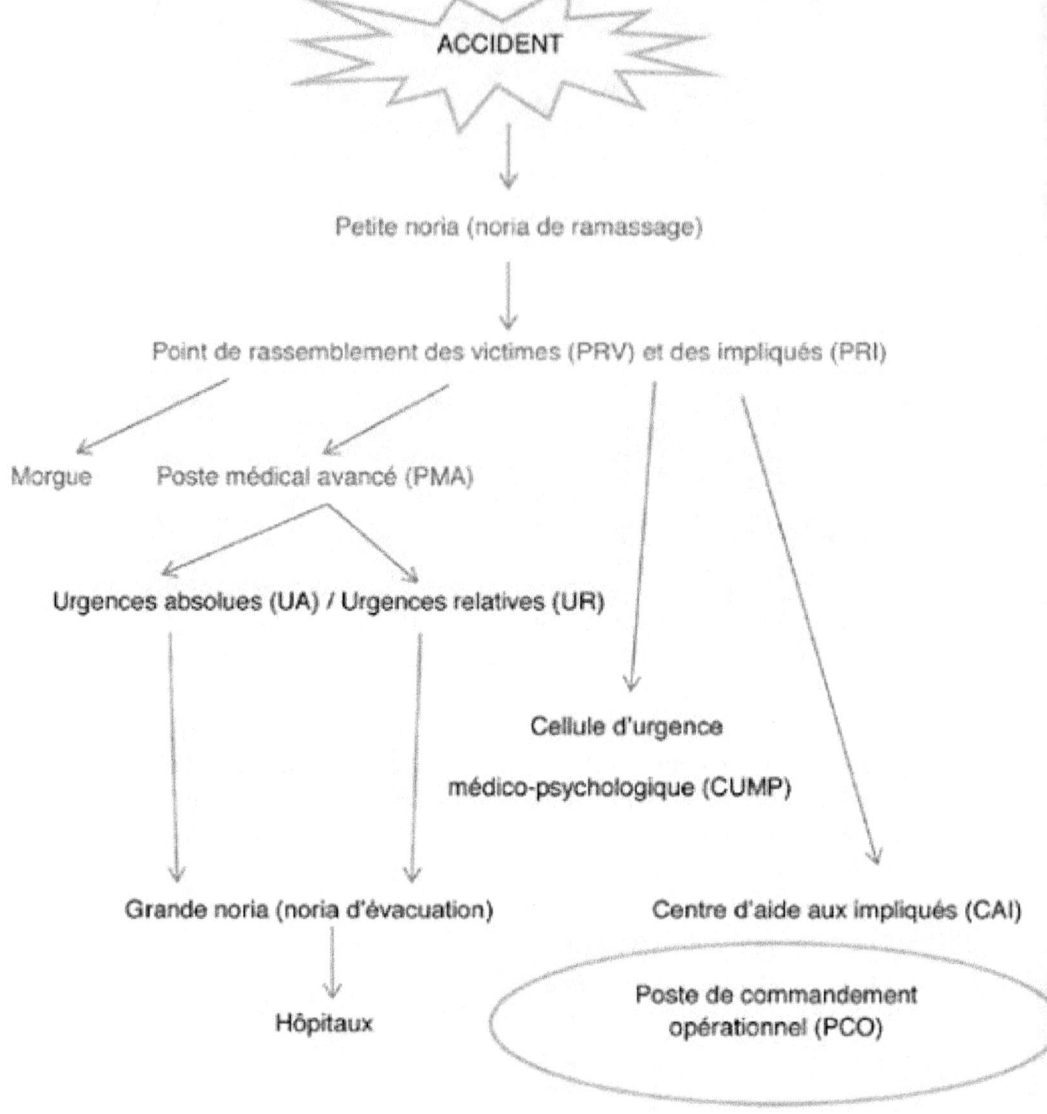

Upon arriving on the scene, make sure to be in a secure area. Park the ambulance so that it does not interfere with the movement of other vehicles and that it can leave quickly, in theory in spur at the side of the other.

Present themselves at the command post (PC): We are usually solicited in LDCS and/or to the great noria. Well stay in complete team and ensure the hardware. The LDCS close to the scene of the accident may be installed in a location requisitioned (coffee, school...) or well under a tent laid down in this use is located in the health posts mobile (PSM 1 or 2) which are equipped with the UAS.
If the accident presents a risk nuclear, radiological, bacteriological, chemical, explosion (NRBC e), the victims and the involved must be decontaminated between the PRV and the LDCS. To participate in the chain of decontamination, it must have held slight of decontamination (TLD), light combinations of decontamination (CLD) or held Overseas (TOM) and have completed the necessary training in their use.
• In LDCS has place the sort of medical emergencies absolute (UA) :
 Extreme - Emergencies (had) : danger of immediate death in the 5 to 15 minutes (rescue of human life);
- First Emergency (U1) : Serious Injuries whose life is not in danger (treatment medico-surgical within 6 hours).

• Then Come emergencies relating (UR) :
- Second Emergency (U2) : serious injuries, treatment of surgical lesions in the 12 to 24 hours;

- Third Emergency (U3) : light injuries.
• Then emergencies exceeded, the involved and the aspect medico-psychological (CUMP: cell of emergency medico-psychological).
All the victims are equipped of a bracelet to bar code and of a medical card of the front (FMA): The **system of digital information standardized (Sinus)** fiabilise the escalation and the treatment of information essential for the follow -up of victims. The bracelet includes barcodes additional stickers to defer on the FMA and all documents or business related to the victim.
Finally it is necessary to know that the first medical team arrived on the scene of the accident provides the direction of medical relief before the arrival of the DSM, made a quick recognition with the DSIS, assesses the number and the state of the victims, fixed the PRV, gives an assessment of the atmosphere at the doctor regulator

of the UAS and determines the location of the LDCS. It does therefore not of victim support.

Memo 142

Digital information system (standardized sinus)

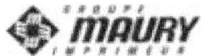

www.ingramcontent.com/pod-product-compliance
Lightning Source LLC
Chambersburg PA
CBHW060819170526
45158CB00001B/25